the Handbag Book of Diet Emergencies

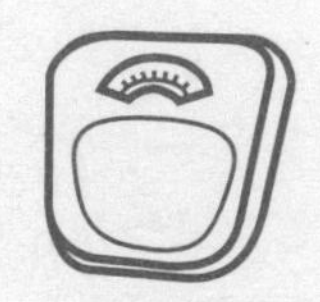

First published in 2004

1 3 5 7 9 10 8 6 4 2

First published by Ebury Press
Random House · 20 Vauxhall Bridge Road · London SW1V 2SA

Random House Australia (Pty) Limited
20 Alfred Street · Milsons Point · Sydney · New South Wales 2061 · Australia

Random House New Zealand Limited
18 Poland Road · Glenfield · Auckland 10 · New Zealand

Random House South Africa (Pty) Limited
Endulini · 5A Jubilee Road · Parktown 2193 · South Africa

Random House UK Limited Reg. No. 954009

www.randomhouse.co.uk

A CIP catalogue record for this book is available from the British Library.

Design by Lovelock and Co

ISBN 0091895979

Papers used by Ebury Press are natural, recyclable products made from wood grown in sustainable forests.

the Handbag Book of Diet Emergencies

Jacqueline Williams

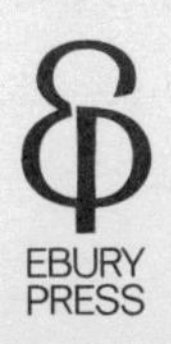

Contents

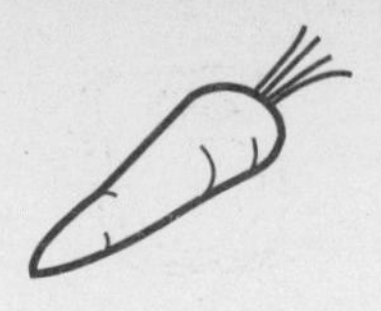

The thing about being on a diet is that you tend to focus on the food you're not 'allowed' to eat and how hungry you feel. It's enough to drive you mad: everywhere you look there are cakes, croissants, buns and bars of chocolate, just begging to be eaten.

So what really works? What will really help you to lose weight, not just today but the whole year and the year after – permanently in fact? Apart from tying yourself up, taping over your mouth or moving to an area of famine – after all it is only our prosperity that makes overeating an option – there are less drastic things that you can do.

What works is you choosing to change your life: choosing healthy food over fast food. Choosing the sorbet or fruit for pudding more often than you have the rich, death-by-chocolate pud. Drinking water instead of fizzy drinks. Making home-made thick-cut chips instead of pre-packaged french fries. Having two pieces of chocolate after dinner instead of the whole bar. Behind every good diet plan, the bottom line is calories – how much you

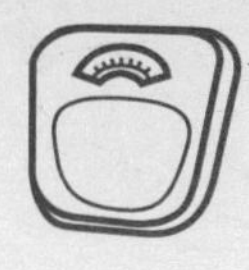

take in determines whether you are overweight or not. It is really that simple. What type of food you eat determines how good you feel, so if you eat health-giving food that's what you'll get.

Food shouldn't equal guilt. Some food is better for you than others. Some foods are more fattening than other foods. At first it will feel unnatural when you can't reach for your favourite food but like learning a new job or riding a bike you'll get the hang of it eventually and it will feel completely natural. The aim is to feel good about food; if you feel bad about eating or restrict it too much you may fall into a cycle of pigging out (bingeing), feeling bad.

Make eating well a lifestyle thing, incorporate some exercise into your life and – before you know it – you're not on a diet, you're living a life where you eat better food and you're at your ideal weight for keeps!

Food is wonderful; it is to be enjoyed, not restricted and obsessed over.

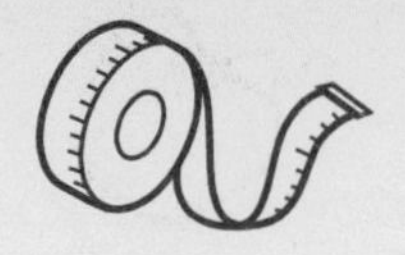

The first thing to do is to make a huge long list of all the foods that you can eat. That's what is important after all, rather than the things you can't have. Put the list where you'll see it every day to remind yourself that there is an abundance of food that you can eat every day. You're not going to go hungry!

The *Handbag Book of Diet Emergencies* is a no-hunger, no-giving-yourself-a-hard-time book. Throw away your control pants – food is your friend.

Warning: This book is not for anybody who wants to keep on feeling guilty about food or people who are skinny but think they are overweight (trust your family and friends on that one) ...

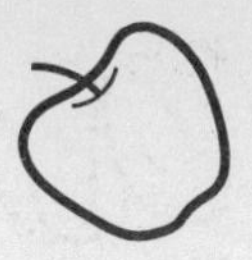

The Girly Emergency Diet

The girly emergency diet – or the *realism* diet – is a mixture of watching the fats, ditching the junk, the sweets and the refined carbs, taking some exercise, and generally sorting out your mind so that you end up with the body you want.

No guilt, no shame, just doing *positive* stuff to make changes.

It is about being *realistic*:

- How much are you prepared to change the way you eat, what are you prepared to give up?
- How much time are you willing to commit to exercise?
- How much do you really want to change your appearance?

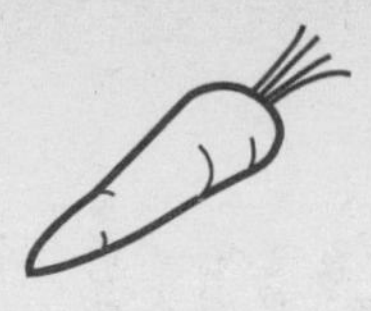

Be honest, and realistic: if you are a big build then you'll never be a size 8 – aim for a size 12 and see what happens.

If you're prepared to make big changes then you can aim high. You make your own rules with the idea that you're then more likely to follow them. Make sure you have enough to eat, but don't keep on eating until you are stuffed and bloated. And give yourself a day off each week where you don't worry overly about what you eat, but don't stuff yourself with rubbish food either.

You and Food

What is your weakness?

If you are going to tackle your weight problem then it is useful to know exactly what your food weaknesses are.

The food test:

1 Would you happily eat pudding in preference to savoury things when you're choosing at the buffet table?

2 Do you get fidgety and cross if you can't get to the shop to buy your chocolate fix?

3 Can you remember a day when you went without chocolate?

4 Have you ever eaten a whole (family-size) chocolate bar or packet of biscuits in one go?

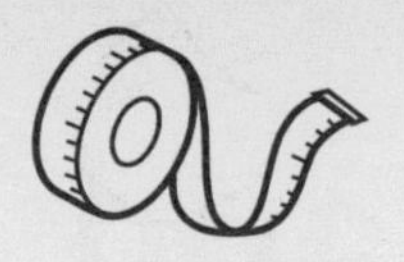

5 If you have a bad day do you dive for a chocolate bar, or do you go for other food?

6 Does tea or coffee also mean chocolate or biscuit to you?

7 Do you always like to eat until really full, practically bursting?

8 Do you eat fast food more than once a week?

9 Is your idea of a supermarket shop a frozen pizza, a couple of boxes of ready meals, pasta, ready-made pasta sauce, biscuits, chocolate, cheese and wine?

10 Do you have a can or more of fizzy drink each day?

11 Do you 'have' to eat a packet of crisps with your sandwich at lunchtime?

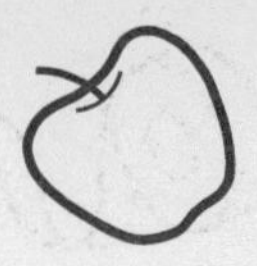

Answers:

If you answered **yes** to all of these questions then it's a wonder you haven't had a heart attack already! You need to seriously rethink your diet.

If you answered **yes** to numbers 1 to 6 sugar is your problem. The problem with eating sugar is that it makes you want to eat even more and that's not just obvious sugars like chocolate, etc. Pasta and refined flour products all raise your blood sugar levels.

If you answered **yes** to 7 to 11 then over-processed and junk food is your problem. The trouble with this food is that there are so many hidden ingredients: sugar, salt and bad fats are just a few of the nasties. You can still eat the same food – but home-cooked so that you get back into the habit of nourishing, additive-free cooking and eating. For example, a simple pizza made at home with mozzarella cheese, tomato sauce and mushrooms will contain a lot less fat and salt than a shop-bought one.

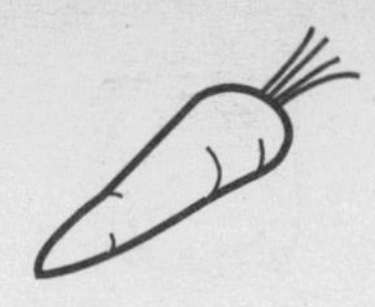

If you have to have it, look at *healthy* ready-prepared food: fresh soups from the supermarket cold cabinet are ideal. But fizzy drinks and crisps will have to be a thing of the past.

We know what we need to do in order to lose weight. The challenge for us all is not to consume excessive calories. We need to eat enough for our needs and then exercise too. Call it a diet if you want to but it works. And it shouldn't be a temporary measure but a way of life.

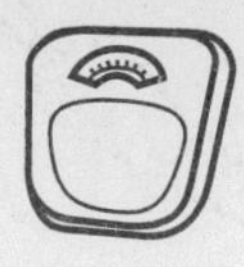

The food you're 'allowed' to eat on a diet is so boring – I'll miss nice food so much ...

Get hold of some new recipes or learn how to cook a wider variety of food so that you don't get bored. And make what you eat strong in flavour.

Thai food has really intense flavours, with fab flavoured seasonings and herbs such as fish sauce, shrimp paste, lime juice, coriander, chilli and ginger which you can cook with chicken and fish.

Japanese is perfect: it's healthy and not high in calories and fat. As long as you stick to sushi or needles and leave the tempura.

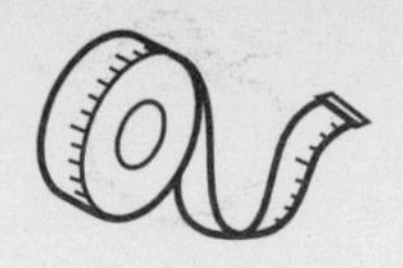

Everyone's banging on about the side effects of diets, it makes me just want to forget losing weight ...

There's loads of talk about the side effects of certain popular diets, particularly the Atkins Diet, although new research has shown that it does work.

You do have to be really careful not to lose weight too quickly. Find a way of eating that suits your life as it is much harder to stick to someone else's idea of what you should eat.

As far as side effects go, one thing is for sure: the side effects of losing weight and eating less junk will be:
clearer skin, easing of PMT symptoms, feeling fitter, increased confidence, more attention from men, a flatter tummy and more choice in clothes, a perkier libido and more energy because you'll be eating better food.

Need we say more?

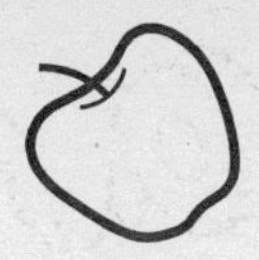

The food diary – facing the truth

Try keeping a food diary and you'll be surprised at how much you really eat: there'll be loads of things you'd have forgotten if you hadn't written them down. Studies show that overweight people underestimate their calorie intake – that is, they think they're eating much less than they really are.

It's not just what you eat but also why you eat it that is interesting to note. When you reach for food that you know you really shouldn't eat but your body craves, note down how you were feeling at the time.

You may be able to think up another solution. For instance, the boss shouts at you, you reach for a chocolate bar. It might be better for your self-esteem and your figure if you were to sort out the problem with your boss instead of soothing yourself with food. Stand up to your boss or get a job where you're happier.

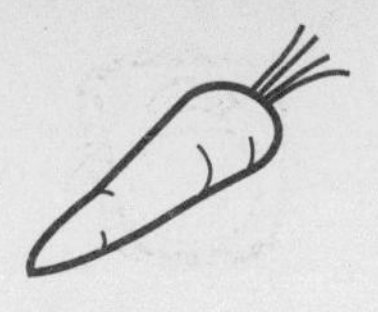

Won't I have to starve myself if I want to lose weight?

You have to reduce your intake of calories which is different from saying reduce your intake of food (that is unless you are gorging yourself all day long).

Even just altering your meal slightly will make a difference: for instance at dinner – instead of a whole plate of pasta with a creamy bacon sauce, have the pasta with tomato sauce.

Your plate should be 1/3 full of vegetables. You'll feel full up because you've had the same bulk of food, but without the calories – and you'll be healthier too with all that veg.

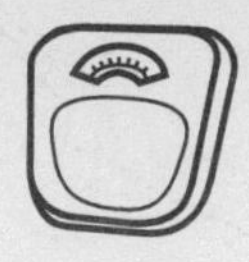

Fast food speeds to your hips

A burger (500 cals) and regular fries (200–400) for lunch is equal to half a day's intake of calories in one meal, and that's before you add drinks and snacks, breakfast and dinner. Have a milkshake with your burger and, at 250+ calories for a small shake, you're really pushing it, with a total of 1000+ calories.

If you're trying to stick to a 1200-calorie diet you'll only have 200 calories left for the day.

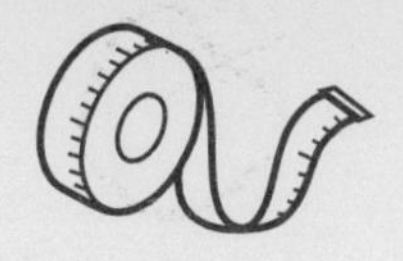

What will I do without chips – they're my favourite.

You can still have them on your pig-out day – make them yourself, by cutting them thickly and frying them in clean oil (oil you haven't used before). Thin french fries absorb more oil than thick-cut ones. Don't buy them out unless you know the chippie is a really good one – the oil used repeatedly in fish and chip shops is so bad for you. Avoid the fast-food french fries, they may seem thin and harmless but they're saturated in oil.

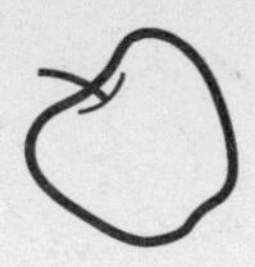

I seriously do not overeat so why am I putting on weight?

Think about where you might be getting calories from, things you might not necessarily think of as food.

- booze – a huge source of calories
- sugar in your tea – 50g (approx 10 spoonfuls) is almost 200 calories, so if you have 5 cups of tea or coffee a day with 2 sugars that is 200 calories just in your tea
- salt – there is hidden salt everywhere, for instance in cheese, salami, ham and bacon, which makes you retain fluid
- sweets – basically just sugar but you might not count them as food
- margarine and butter – do you pile it on? A scraping will still make your toast or sandwich tasty. Or if the bread is really delicious go without, and enjoy the flavour of the bread

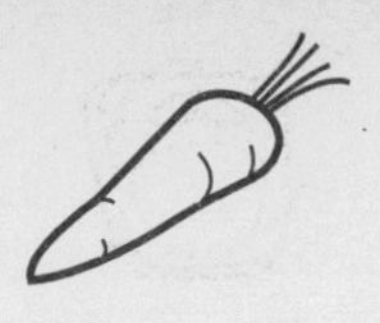

Snack Attack

- Snacking properly will actually help you to lose weight – it keeps blood sugar levels steady and stops you needing a sugar hit.

- The trick is to snack healthily before you get the urge for something sweet.

How much do you really eat?

A recent study showed that people who are overweight underestimate how much they eat. Could that be you? Try keeping a food diary to find out how much you really do eat (see page 17).

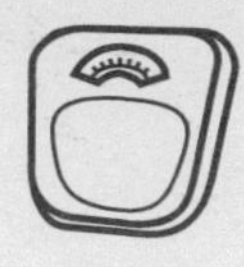

Top tips for bringing down the calorie count

- Nachos and cheese 608 cal – burritos, beans and cheese 378. A lot less cals and the burritos are much more of a meal and comfort food than nachos
- Make your dips with yoghurt instead of cream
- Choose the hummus dip instead of taramasalata
- Avoid Greek-style yoghurt (its creaminess should give it away) – it is about 5 times higher in fat than other full-fat yoghurts

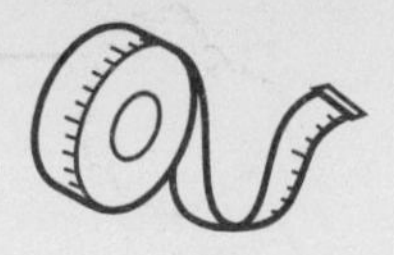

Watching what I eat is so difficult, can't you suggest some easy things to give up?

Surely you can give up your daily OJ? If you have it every morning you'd quickly get through a litre, which is equal to about 375 calories. Drink water instead and you can have that 375 cals in food instead.

The calories saved would allow you to have a weekly croissant. That's great news.

Or you can leave off those calories, to help you reach your ideal weight faster.

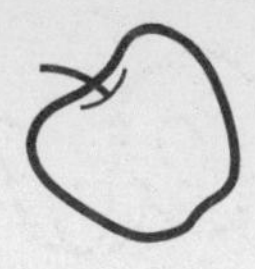

I feel really unhappy and deprived if I'm not full after a meal.

Believe it or not, eating protein (fat) gives you a more satisfied, full feeling for much longer after eating.

Eating protein foods instead of a plate of pasta should stop you from falling off the healthy-eating wagon. Eating a carbohydrate meal often means you need to eat more to feel full.

The hugely popular Atkins Diet works on this principle: you cut down on the carbs and eat more fat. It might not be perfect in every way but I don't know anyone who ever went hungry on this diet.

Among the carb foods, choose carefully – go for foods that are digested more slowly like brown rather than white rice, wholewheat bread instead of white. But avoid foods that raise your blood sugar level; once this dips again you can feel weak and hungry and go reaching for more food, usually a weight-gaining carbohydrate.

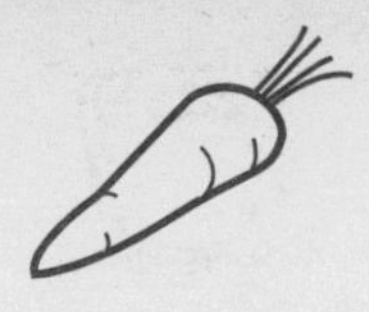

Afternoon snack attack

Eating protein for lunch can help you feel fuller and more satisfied and you will probably then get by with fruit for a snack rather than chocolate.

- Good sources of protein for lunch: tuna sandwich (brown bread), chicken salad, ham and cheese quiche, salmon, omelette. Most of the supermarkets do good-quality, prepacked meals with these foods in them.

- Eating pasta for lunch will make you feel full and satisfied at first. Your blood sugar levels will soar and then when they come crashing down again you'll feel tired, bloated and hanging out for a sweet afternoon snack.

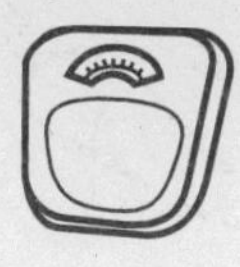

Help, I can't live without chocolate.

Chocolate makes you feel good, that's true, so look for ways you can get the feel-good effect elsewhere.

- Grab your man for a romp – no, this is not an excuse to shag some other guy if yours isn't handy. 'I didn't mean to sleep with him, I was just dying for some chocolate' won't wash I'm afraid.

OR

- Go for a run, you'll get the same euphoric high but without the guilt. To satisfy your taste buds craving for something sweet, demolish some dried or fresh fruit with a large glass of water.

- If you are really desperate for chocolate, make yourself run to the furthest shop from your house to buy it. Run home again before unwrapping and eating. Enjoy it.

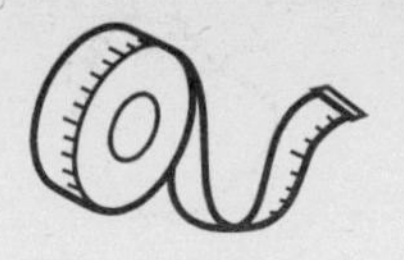

Healthy chocolate treat

After all that nagging I'll let you in on the good news about chocolate:
A good-quality dark chocolate (it must be at least 70% cocoa) contains antioxidant ingredients which prevent fats in the blood from clogging the arteries.

Smoothies to fill you up

If a salad or a sandwich isn't enough to fill you up at lunch time then have a smoothie made with soya milk or low-fat milk, with fruit and a tablespoon of yoghurt. Drink it slowly and it'll feel like a meal in itself.

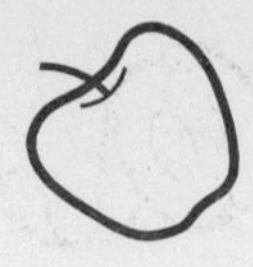

It's not fair, I'm stuck with a slow metabolism; my mates fill their faces non-stop with stuff I daren't eat and I'm still twice their size. How can I speed up my metabolism?

Are you sure that it's a case of fast and slow metabolism? Maybe you only see your mates when they pig out and usually they eat quite sensibly. Are you completely honest about what you eat, sometimes people who think they eat nothing blank out a fair bit of what they eat – take the food test on page 11.

Life is unfair, it's a sad fact. Some people do seem to get away with eating a huge amount. Counting and controlling calories is more important for people whose bodies are more inclined to store excess fat as energy rather than flushing it through.

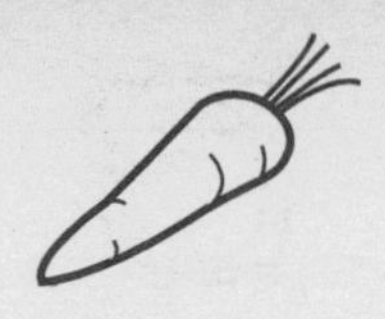

Metabolism

The bad news: your metabolism slows as you get older.

The good news: if you get into good habits – and good shape – now you'll have it sorted for life.

Girly bum barometer

Feel like your bum is growing out of all proportion to the rest of your body? Is it bigger than it's ever been?

Ask your best workmate which other woman in the office has a bum most like yours in size and shape and watch it. Watch it bounce about and generally look too big.

That bum is your motivation for exercising and sorting yours out. Today.

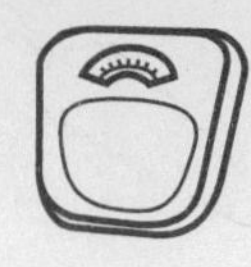

Help, I'm always hungry!

- If you must graze, make sure it's on healthy snacks. Chop up an apple into small pieces so that it takes longer to eat. Have carrots handy. Doesn't sound very exciting?

- Try eating larger portions (of the right foods) at mealtimes so that you're not hungry soon after. And don't eat foods that cause rapid fluctuations in your blood sugar levels – this will cause further sugar cravings.

- Good (complex) carbs take longer to be absorbed by the body and so don't raise your blood sugar levels in the same way as simple carbs. They include wholewheat bread and pasta, brown rice, and veg.

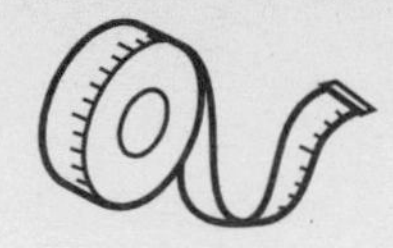

I always start my diet with the best intentions and then I blow it by stuffing down a whole packet of biscuits or a family-sized bag of crisps.

Give yourself a day off each week when you can eat your junk treats. Sunday is a good one as you've got time on your hands and you might be feeling fragile from a late and boozy Saturday night.

Feel like going on a binge? Adopt the AA approach:

- phone a friend
- go for a walk
- drink something non-fattening
- have sex
- take up knitting
- buy yourself flowers instead of a bag of buns/donuts

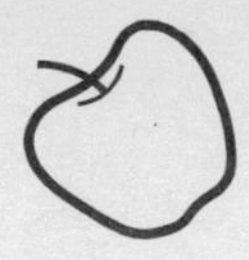

Snacking is an art form

(get it right and you're less likely to reach for a chocolate bar or ten)

Try:

- raw nuts such as cashews
- fresh fruit – cut it up and make it a treat
- a smoothie
- rice cakes with banana or avacado on top
- wholegrain bread toasty snacks: make them elaborate and extravagant – combine all your favourite foods on one cracker. (Mine is weird but gorgeous – a little Branston pickle on the bottom, ricotta cheese then slices of apple – a quick toast under the grill and then add alfalfa sprouts. You might gag but you'll discover these mad combos when you're trying to find quick and tasty snack food.)

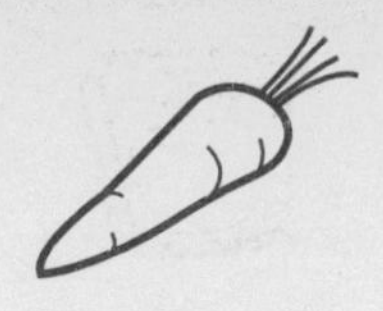

Your friends (fat within/thin without!)

- oily fish
- extra-virgin olive oil
- avocados, nuts and seeds

(Such foods, high in health-giving fat, have been shown to help ward off heart disease, depression, some cancers and dry-skin complaints.)

Your main enemies

- sugar
- chocolate
- fizzy drinks
- sweets
- crisps
- eating in front of the telly
- bowl after bowl of pasta – eat sensible portions
- second helpings at every meal
- eating until way after full-up point
- any fast food
- salt – it can make you retain water which can be up to 3 lbs in weight

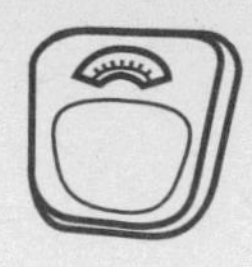

Is there something wrong with me? It doesn't seem fair that I can be on the same diet as a friend and they'll be the one who loses weight and I don't.

Sadly some people are more prone to putting on weight than others. If you and a friend eat identical meals, your friend might not draw as much nutrient from the food and get rid of the excess while you might store it as fat.

The person who loses their excess calories in the loo would have a tougher time surviving if food were in short supply. Their system is not as efficient at storing food as fat for when they might need it.

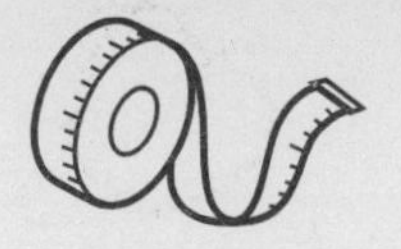

Fat-free misery

Be careful buying fat-free or low-fat food.

Fat-free food can be loaded with sugar and it doesn't satisfy and fill you up as much as full-fat food does.

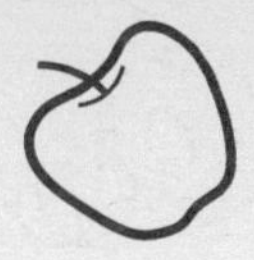

Comfort for bad days

- a big bowl of mashed potato – fry some onions in olive oil for about 10 mins and sprinkle on the top
- go to bed – sleeping burns off 60 calories an hour
- a vodka cocktail is relatively low in calories – have several with your mates
- shopping for two hours is equivalent to an hour's walk but not if you spend all of your time in the changing rooms (240 an hour)
- if it's sale time and you're dashing about trying to find a bargain you could burn up to 360 cals an hour
- go for a float at your local swimming pool – you might end up doing some laps – you might not. Enjoy the water
- bake a cake and invite your mates to share it

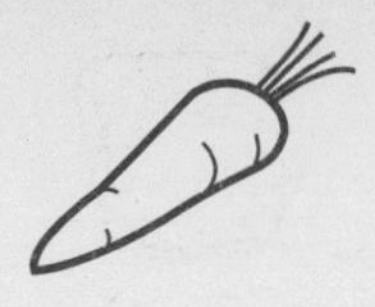

The truth about cellulite

Help – I have seriously orange peel-dimpled cellulite on my bum and the back of my thighs – what can I do to shift it?

Cellulite is fat; lumpy, irregular fat deposits to be more precise. It's that it happens to be on your arse that makes it a more emotive issue. OK, if it was on your arms it wouldn't be a good look either but we are all especially sensitive about our bums.

Every woman can fall prey to it: if it's any comfort skinny girls get it too. Anti-cellulite treatments and diets abound but what is the truth about cellulite?

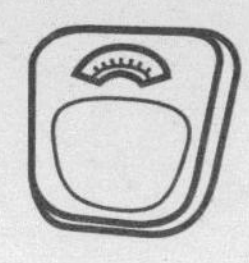

The myth:

Cellulite is trapped toxins – give up coffee, alcohol and chocolate, and drink lots of water to flush out the toxins.

Fact:

Chubby babies have cellulite – do you think that they have done something to 'deserve' it. Eaten too many toxins? I don't think so.

The confusion:

Some experts claim that cellulite is a fluid-retention problem and so drinking more water as we're all told to do can actually make it worse.

We're told coffee is a toxin that we must give up but then we're told that a cup of coffee boosts your metabolism and helps circulation.

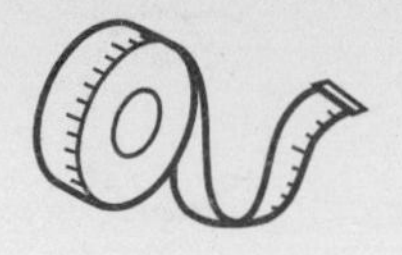

What really helps:

One thing that is bound to help is improving your circulation. Yoga is the perfect exercise for doing this. Madonna got back her pre-baby body with Ashtanga yoga. Demi Moore also practises it and she has recently overhauled her body for the *Charlie's Angels* film. Gwyneth Paltrow is always snapped with her yoga mat on the way to a class and she always looks fit and healthy.

Massage, body brushing and decreasing your intake of salt to reduce water retention should all help improve the appearance of cellulite-troubled areas.

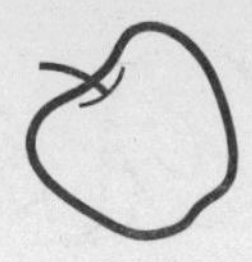

I've just completely blown it – my diet has been going so well and then I ate a whole packet of biscuits and two chocolate bars.

Oooh, what sort were they? Oops!

It happens, don't give yourself a hard time about it. Getting upset and feeling ashamed are only going to make things worse. Move on!

It's worth thinking about what led to the binge – an emotional upset, boredom, or an irresistible display of cakes. Cheer yourself up in another way that doesn't involve food. Or have a good long look at the display and then walk on by. Deal with the issue that led to the binge and you're a long way towards preventing it from happening again.

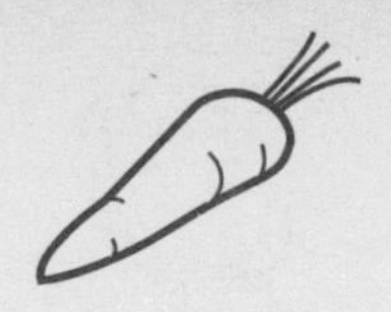

Girly get a grip

Massage belts, saunas, wraps.
You will lose weight but they don't really work to keep weight off. Saunas and wraps don't melt fat but make you lose fluid.

Which is fine – you will keep the weight off if you plan never to drink anything, ever again!

The Jennifer Lopez look

Accept your pear shape if you are slim elsewhere. Shaping up is the thing: exercise to get your legs, bum and hips in great shape.

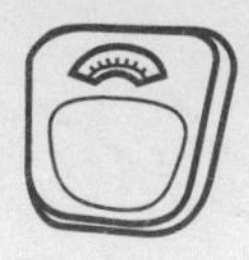

I need to lose weight fast – will slimming foods help?

Probably not and ...

- they're expensive
- they can make you constipated – and sometimes contain laxative to counteract that problem
- lots of artificial substitutes are used – yuk!
- is a chalky milkshake your idea of food?

Girly beware of

- Any 'diet' or low-fat foods that warn of laxative effect
- Low-fat food that is loaded with sugar

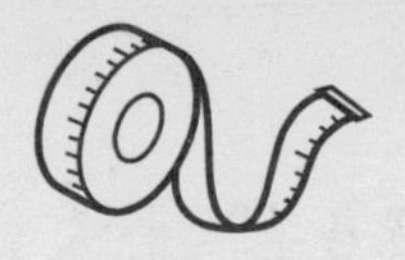

Girly Golden Rules

- Always have a snack with you wherever you go
- No second helpings
- Don't lie to yourself about what you eat
- Eat and enjoy – don't watch telly or read – concentrate on every mouthful
- Don't visit friends who live on junk
- Accept the truth – your weight really is about what food, and how much, goes into your body
- Eat 3 meals a day
- Don't let yourself get over-hungry
- Have food at home, in your handbag, in your desk drawer
- Never shop when you're hungry
- Forget yo-yo dieting
- Keep it simple – eat less junk and more good stuff and get off your arse and get physical

Your Body

Dressing to conceal or reveal

Help, I've put on a stone; I've got a really cool party coming up – what can I wear?

If you've put on weight, chances are your boobs are bigger too, so wear

- clothes that put your chest in the limelight and your ass in the shade. Try a V-neck dress or a black strappy top with flattering, fitting trousers, also in a dark colour
- a trouser suit with a jacket cut long to cover bulgy bits but don't wear anything underneath except a cleavage-enhancing bra. Wear a choker or necklace to draw attention to your neck and cleavage and get on out there

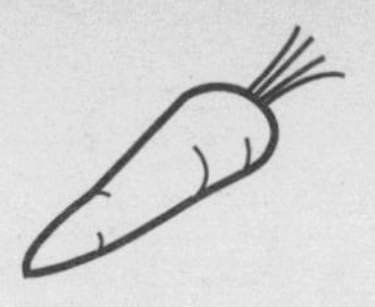

Help, I've gone up a size, what to do?

Well either hold on and don't buy anything until you've slimmed down, or buy the right size. Nothing is more bulge-inducing than wearing clothes and underwear that are too small or too tight.

Even small women can make this mistake and it looks awful.

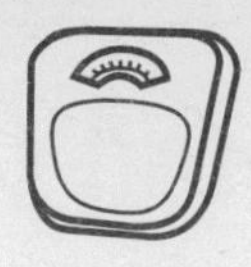

I've got a glam party coming up and I want to look really fab ...

- Most of us are pretty good at sorting out our outerwear but often the thing we forget or leave till the last minute is finding the right underwear.

- Good underwear is key – so many times you'll see a woman who looks fab but she has bulges around her bra strap and knicker line. Take your outfit with you when you buy the underwear and try it on.

- Be honest about your body and wear something that really highlights the best bits.

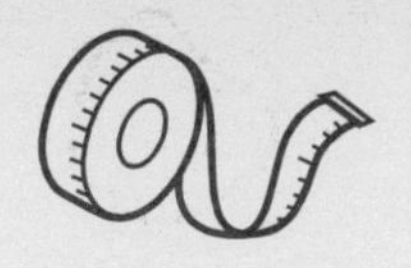

Nightmare, I've put on weight since I last wore my favourite trouser suit. What are the best knickers for keeping my bulges under control?

Control pants are the answer! They're not exactly sexy but they're fab, brilliantly effective in a pot-belly emergency.

Trinny and Susannah swear by Magic Shorts by Bodie and Gibbs (BodieandGibbs.co.uk). They're guaranteed to disguise bums and tums that need a little … reining in, shall we say …

Girdles A bit restrictive in the main but if you shop around you might find one that's bearable. Try the big department stores as well as specialist bra and underwear fitters.

Corsets Can be really sexy and definitely tummy tucking. Try some of the chains like La Sensa and Anne Summers for sexy and toning corsets.

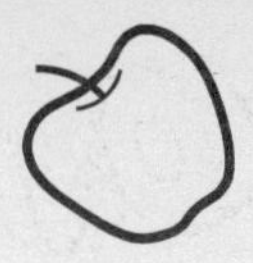

Appearance tricks

- pot belly – throw back your shoulders, stand up straight, look straight ahead. Don't sag into your middle when standing or sitting, or you will accentuate your pot
- big bum – go for the brazen J-Lo effect, wear long cardigans that skim your bottom, or forget trousers and wear skirts
- chunky legs – choose skirts or wide-legged but well-fitting trousers. If you're really self-conscious wear a long – but not baggy – cardigan
- big arms – wear sleeves if they're wobbly, or get into the gym and tone them up
- double chin – your posture is important; don't slump in your seat, walk tall and keep your head up

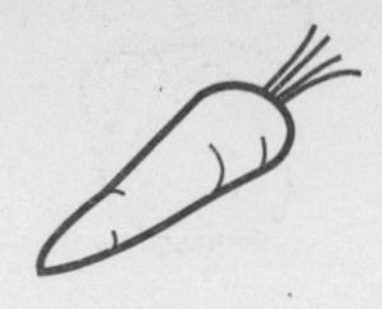

Will baggy clothes hide the extra weight I'm carrying?

Often they'll just make you look bigger than you are. If you buy well-shaped clothes you'll look much sleeker. You can look good in fitted trousers and tops rather than flowing tent-like tops. Baggy clothes will just make you look ... er ... baggy.

Even if you're fed up that you've gone up a size, don't be tempted to buy a size too small; you won't fool anybody and your bulges will just be more noticeable.

Girly bulge checklist

- bras – must fit around your back otherwise you'll have bulges above and below the straps
- pants – even skinny birds get bulges if the elastic is in the wrong places. When you find a flattering fit – buy lots of pairs
- shirts – if the buttons gape don't wear it, it will draw attention to the fact that you're bursting out

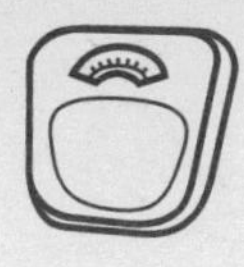

Help, I feel huge – how will I ever get a pair of jeans to fit me?

Shop around, there are so many different styles to choose from. Marks and Gap have a huge range. Or try a department store where they'll bring lots of different styles to you in the changing rooms. Choose carefully and you will find the right pair.

- Large front pockets will shorten your legs so avoid them unless you're tall
- Small front pockets will make your bum look bigger. Stay away if you want your bum to look small. Great if your waist is your trouble spot
- Low-waisted jeans will let any belly flab hang out – and watch out when you sit down or you'll look like Michelin woman
- If you have a big stomach, high waistbands will make your tummy look bigger so go for a waistband in between a high waist and hipsters

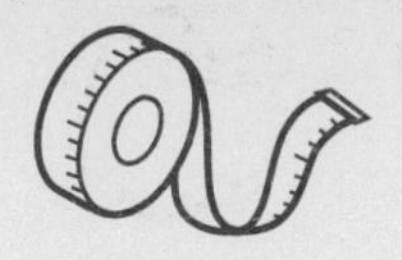

I've got a pot belly and I really want to wear a slinky dress for a big night out.

Control pants – they ain't sexy to look at but they'll tame your bumps and make you look sexy on the outside. Go to a department store where they have those nice middle-aged ladies who've seen every body-shape there is. They won't be snooty and they'll get you exactly what you need.

Or you could try a good old-fashioned girdle. As well as pulling everything in it stops that hideous indentation line you get from your underwear when you're carrying a bit of extra weight.

Okay so they're not ideal and certainly not the sexiest thing in the world but it's a special occasion and think how good you'll look in the photos!

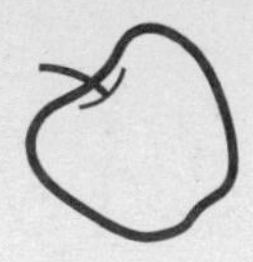

I'll do anything to get a flat tummy.

Avoid excess salt, it causes your body to retain fluid. Think about the salty things you eat. Most of us eat too many crisps, nuts and other similar snacks, Chinese, pizza, salami, ham and other processed meats. What happens is that water is retained until your kidneys are able to clear the excess fluid, which is why you puff up.

Go easy on beans, pulses, cereal and dairy products.

Eat soups where you know little salt has been added.

Fish, rice and salads will all help you keep a flat tummy.

Chew well and don't rush or gulp your food.

Avoid fizzy mineral water, beer and fizzy drinks.

Watch your intake of bread, cheese and anything else containing yeast.

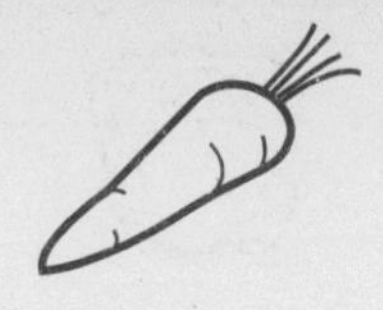

I hate going shopping, I can't ever seem to find anything to fit me, it's so depressing ...

Sorry but you need to get out there and try again. This is a problem for all girls from time to time, not just bigger ones. You need to find the store that's right for you. It may change from season to season or you might be lucky and they'll always have things in the right shape and size for you.

The girls who look their best all of the time are the ones who shop and shop: to find the styles, colours and labels that suit them.

Ask anyone you know who has a similar shape to you where they get their clothes from. Don't worry, there will be a shop to suit you. Or you could try posting your problem on a website like handbag.com.

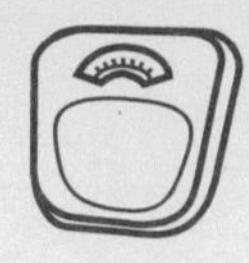

I weigh myself every day but it seems to vary wildly; sometimes it goes up after days and days of being really good!

Remember the Special K ad where the woman puts on a red dress that's she's had for years and it still fits (supposedly because she's been eating Special K)?

Well, having a weight-testing clingy outfit is a really good idea for checking how you're going with your size. Choose a dress that is close-fitting, either Lycra-ish or with a zip. Whether or not the dress fits is a much more reliable test than jumping on the scales every day.

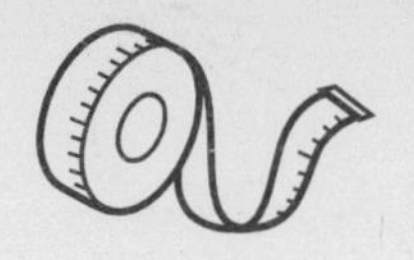

Oh God! I'm usually a size 12 but I seem to have ballooned to size 14, though I really don't think I've put that much weight on ...

Don't panic, the truth is that sizes vary wildly from store to store and also between brands. You might be a 12 in Oasis but a 14 in Top Shop. The size you take in the same shop can also vary from season to season depending on styles and cuts.

The ultimate test of if you are expanding or not is if you start bursting out of your fave jeans that you've been wearing for years. Don't ditch them, hang on to them and use them as your weight-gain tester. If they fit, you're doing all right, if not, reconsider your diet and exercise levels.

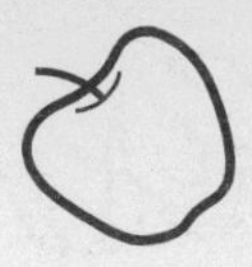

Photoshopping

First find a photo of yourself where you look absolutely stunning apart from looking heavier than you'd like to.

Then, using white-out, paint around your excess curves on hips, thighs, bum and tummy until you get the shape you desire. Pin up the picture where you can see it.

Or if you or a mate has access to Photoshop (a computer programme where it is possible to 'airbrush' photographs) you can do a more sophisticated job of this by scanning the photo and then doing your 'whiteing out' on screen.

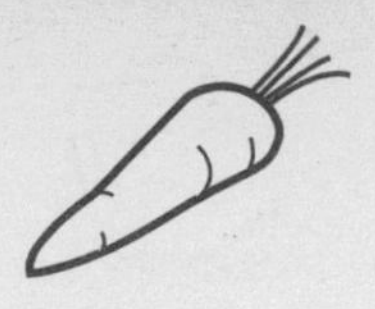

I'm getting married next year and I want to look my absolute best

Most weddings are booked more than a year ahead so you can't really say you haven't had a chance to think about losing weight and getting in shape.

Make a list of the foods you can and can't have. Take up exercise now. Be realistic and don't try and lose too much weight or you might have trouble staying at the same weight between your dress fitting and the actual day.

Losing weight

This is a time when Dr Atkins just might get you to your ideal weight; then you can move on to a less stringent eating plan to keep the weight off.

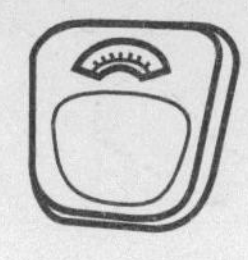

Maintaining your weight

You might use nerves and stress as an excuse for putting on weight leading up to the wedding but don't forget you'll have to live with that wedding album for a long, long time.

When you have your dress fitted make sure somebody takes a photo of you to inspire you to stay the same weight so you'll fit in that dress on the day.

Motivation

Get one of your bridesmaids to exercise with you. Compete with each other to see who can get the fittest and look the most sleek. As the bride, it's your job to get your body into the best shape.

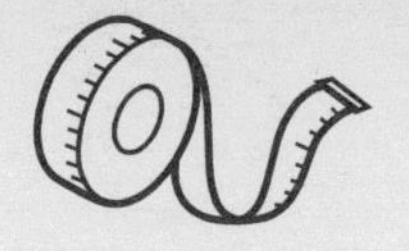

The dress

Try to achieve your ideal weight before your dress fitting, never ever be tempted to get fitted at a smaller size with the intention of dieting into the dress. It is too expensive, and stressful, a risk to take.

If you're buying your dress ready-made then, yes, maybe you can aim for the smaller size. Find the one that you want now and aim to buy the next size down when you've lost the weight. Drive them crazy in the shop by going back for regular try-ons if you think you're losing weight.

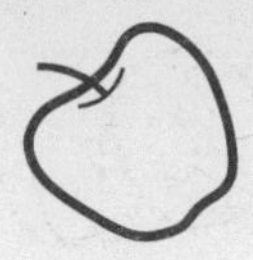

Whether it's for your honeymoon, or your annual holiday in the sun, you need to try before you buy, but . . .

- don't make things worse by trying on clothes under the glaring fluorescent lights of a communal changing room.

- Tell the assistant you don't have time to try them on, buy a range of styles, have a stress-free time trying them on at home and if they don't suit you return them.

- As long as they're in perfect condition and within 14 days of purchase most stores are happy to refund or exchange (check the store policy before you buy).

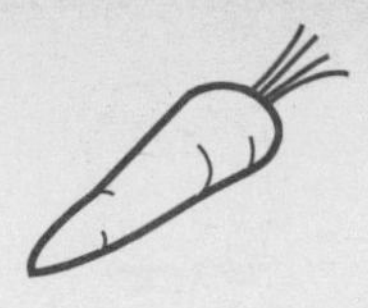

Holidays – daring to bare

Aaghhh – it's spring, and summer hols are fast approaching. I can't face squeezing into a bikini again!

- Do be brave and get last summer's bikini out. Try it on, look in the mirror. How bad is it?
- Don't be a big baby and lose heart, just be real about what you need to do to sort it out. Set yourself a programme. How much do you want to lose? How much exercise can or will you do?
- Console yourself by remembering you'll look so much better once you've done some exercise: at the very least you'll lose a bit of weight and firm up what you've got.
- Get a mate to help you apply an all-over fake tan or pay for an all-over spray job. Now you're ready to face the changing rooms to find a gorgeous new bikini!

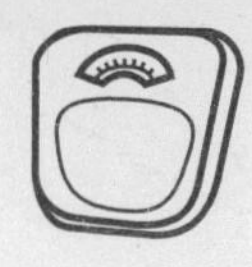

Every year it's the same: I plan to get in shape for my holidays but never quite manage it. Any advice ...?

You can achieve surprisingly good results in a short time.

The holiday countdown:

8 weeks till your holiday – you can achieve good results in this time, 10–16 lbs weight loss with careful eating and exercise. Drink lots of water and eat three good meals a day with a little carb, protein and at least 2/3 of a plate of vegetables.

4 weeks – if you lose 2 lbs a week until you go you're looking at a total loss of 8 lbs, which would make a stunning difference to your bikini look.

2 weeks – you can lose up to 4 lbs by cutting out all sugar and eating carbs only once a day. Firm up your legs and bottom by swimming, so push yourself to go 3–4 times a week.

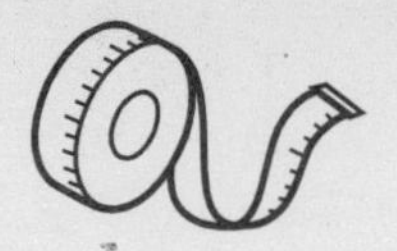

Next week: we're taking a last-minute package deal. Eek, spray on some fake tan, buy a king-size sarong, suck in your belly for the entire holiday and never move too fast or run anywhere, or it will all wobble!

Seriously have a fab holiday and limit yourself to how much you think about how you look. There's no point spending the entire holiday thinking 'I look huge, I'm really fat'. It's a waste of headspace and will ruin your holiday – relax, think about something else, stare into space, read a book, anything except be mean to yourself.

If your problem bits are below the waist: buy a bikini top that accentuates your breasts. Draw eyes to them and away from your problem bits.

Get a matching pair of shorts that cover more of your scary bits than an ordinary pair of bikini pants will. Lots of shops now sell mix-and-match pants and bikini tops so check them out.

Motivation and Self-control

We live in a world of quick fixes and having what we want when we want it, so the idea of giving up food we like – even if it does us no favours – is not a popular one.

We want to be slim but we don't want to have to put ourselves out too much to achieve it. We moan that our bodies – and our lives – aren't as wonderful as celebs and yet we choose to ignore that they often sacrifice a lot to have the bodies they do. Some of the diets and exercise regimes they undertake require them to completely turn their lives upside down, sometimes for months at a time.

Before you protest that you haven't the time or can't be bothered to spend all that time watching what you eat, stop and think. The fact is that many of you devote loads of time and energy to it anyway; most

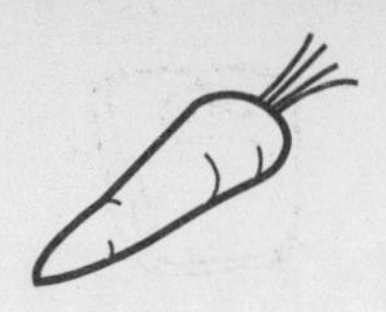

of us spend our lives on diets and waste a lot of time thinking and obsessing about our weight. Always comparing our bodies to others', constantly worrying that we're too fat, never liking our bodies ... All this is time consuming and wearing. Imagine how much more slimmer we'd be if we turned the obsessing and moaning into action.

What it eventually comes down to if you're totally honest with yourself is that it is your choice.

Why you want to lose weight? Can you visualise yourself being slimmer than you are now?

How much would you like to weigh?

It is much more effective to focus on the positive: what you want to be than what you want to lose.

Set yourself weight-loss goals, 2 lbs per week is totally realistic and should get you to the weight you want to be.

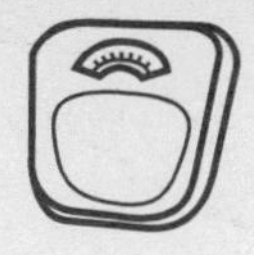

Girly Classic Cons

- I'll start my diet tomorrow (like which tomorrow, 2010?)
- I don't really eat that much (tubs of ice cream eaten in secret do count)
- It's not my fault, it's all those ads for chocolate and junk food (they don't hold you down and shovel it into your mouth though, do they?)
- I'll go to the gym tomorrow (it's today that you want to lose weight though, isn't it?)
- All those skinny chicks in magazines just give a false standard of what size we should be (that's true but this is about you and what you think the right weight is for you – your aim shouldn't be skinny, it should be healthy)

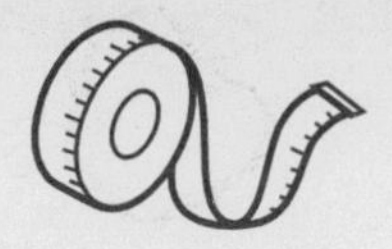

Vulnerable (= danger) times

It helps to know when your weakest times are and how to cope. Plan a strategy for nightmare situations, whenever they arise.

Problem: I got dumped
Usual solution: A whole tub of ice cream
New solution: Same as the old – come on, of course you need it then – but after that, no more comfort eating. Ask a friend around and you'll only eat half the tub

Problem: Broke
Usual solution: Watch a lot of telly and eat crisps
New solution: The ideal time to get your mate out for an evening walk, making it to the pub just before closing time. You can't spend more than the cost of a half, as the bar will close before you finish your drink. And you'll have to walk home too

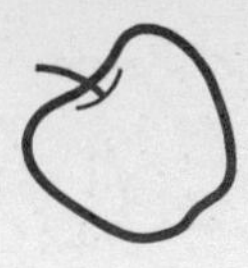

Problem: **Bored**

Usual solution: Raiding the fridge every five minutes

New solution: Ring up all your mates instead. Get yourself an unlimited talk-time package or it will ruin your phone bill. You'll turn into a real gossip head but it'll keep you out of the fridge

Scenario: **Girls' night in**

(danger time for mass choccy/ice cream/crisps feeding event)

Usual solution: Eat it all

New solution: Put in a bit more effort – try and outdo each other by bringing tasty, healthy dips and snacks. Get some exercise too, suggest couch Olympics – have a race jumping from couch to couch. Dance: take your newest CDs. Find a stick and do the limbo – a great pissed-up girly game. A game of Twister will also burn off calories

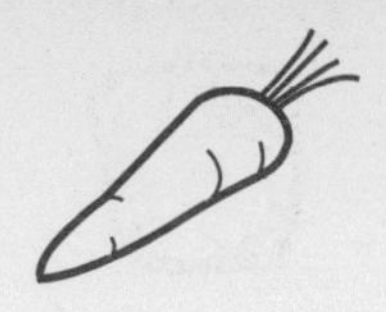

Problem: Wintertime

Usual solution: Eating too many carbs, to keep warm

New solution: Make yourself huge batches of filling soups, eat some with a hunk of wholewheat bread and freeze some. Keep down your intake of carbs

Scenario: Holiday

Usual situation: Pigging out on food and beer, wine and snacks

New solution: choose lighter foods especially seafood and chicken. Eat some bread but not the entire baguette/loaf. Drink wine instead of beer and forget sugary fizzy drinks. This will stop you looking all bloated in your glam, itsy-bitsy bikini

Scenario: Girls' night out

(danger time for crisps with drinks, junk-food at closing time)

Usual situation: Eat it all

Solution: Eat before you go. After closing time go straight home

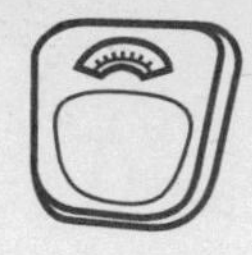

Problem: **Junk-food addict friends**

Usual solution: eat junk too

New solution: You've got to stay away from them, eat before you see them, meet them when they won't be eating or leave them well before they head for McDonald's

Scenario: **Settled relationship – you suddenly become more of a couch potato**

Usual solution: go out to clubs (to get your dancing exercise in) or hanging around in bars (standing around uses up calories too) Suddenly becoming less active can reduce your need for calories by 200–500 per day

New solution: Go for long romantic walks, have loads of sex. Or make the effort to go out dancing or walk to the pub together

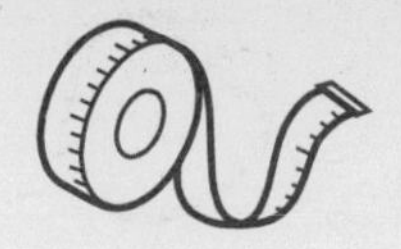

How can I stop myself from dashing to the shop for a Mars bar every afternoon?

Snacking. This isn't a dirty word – your body needs food regularly to keep going. Think of those times when your craving was so intense you had to dash to the shop mid-afternoon for a bar of chocolate. If you'd kept up your intake and not let your blood sugar levels plummet you wouldn't have found yourself craving it. Snack time should be at the same time every day – figure out when you usually get your cravings and make snack time before that to ward off the pangs. You should always have supplies in your desk drawer. Go for a walk at lunchtime a couple of times a week to buy seasonal fruit: bananas, satsumas and oranges in winter; cherries, peaches and strawberries in summer.

If you still find yourself lusting after something sweet, go on an arse-spotting tour of the office. Take in the big ones in all their wobbly glory – that's what your Mars bars will cost you.

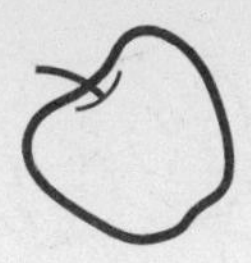

Girly diet sabotage

- birthdays
- weddings
- Friday nights out after a hard week
- rainy days
- hanging out with friends who eat junk
- people who say 'your face was prettier when you were plump'

Give yourself a break!

Have Fridays off (or a weekend day if you find weekends hardest).

Eat some of the treats you crave all week without giving yourself a hard time.

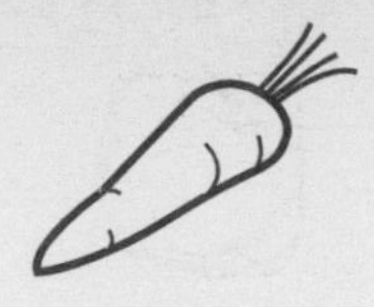

How do I stick to eating well? A bad day sends me back into my old eating habits.

You can bounce back from bad days without caving in entirely, so don't have a tantrum or sink into a depression about it. Be nice to yourself on bad days.

A bad day is just that, a day, so get over it and get on with your new sensible eating lifestyle.

Whatever you do don't starve yourself the next day – just try cutting back a little, 200 cals or so.

Stop!

Next time you feel the urge to overeat, stop and think about what you're about to put in your mouth. Wait 5 minutes and if you still want it then grab your coat and go for a walk.

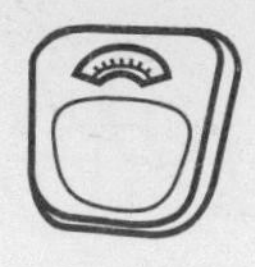

I was doing really well at first, I lost half a stone, but despite eating really carefully that's as much as I seem able to lose. Why have I stopped losing weight?

You've reached a plateau. In some ways this is good news as it often happens after a period of steady weight loss. Your body now needs a chance to get used to your new weight. Basically what has happened is that when you lose weight your body thinks that there is a shortage of food and so tries to conserve energy to hang on to the body mass that you have by slowing down your metabolism.

Weight loss will be slower for a while but don't get fed up; just let your body adjust and then look forward to the next phase. My hunch is that the more time you give your body to adjust, the more likely you are to keep the weight off and find your ideal weight.

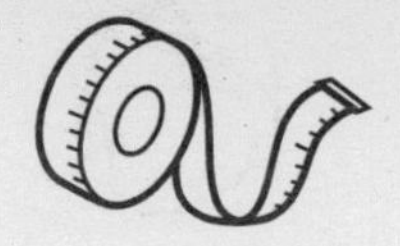

It's normal to:

- put on a little weight in winter (2–4 lbs)
- put on weight in pregnancy (a max. of 22–28 lbs for the entire pregnancy)
- eat too much at Christmas time
- have a day's break each week to pig out a little (not binge)
- have your weight fluctuate – weigh yourself once a month and in the nude
- snack – as long as it's on 'good' food
- eat chocolate or ice cream if your boyfriend dumps you

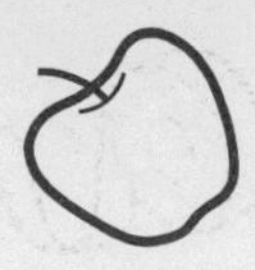

Find a way of eating that suits your lifestyle – many diets are complicated and involve eating in a way that is too hard to fit into your life.

Always in a rush: then think ahead and sort out food to suit. Cook in bulk when you are at home.

Always eating out: make sure you know exactly what it is that you can eat when you go out and choose wisely.

Know which foods and which times of day you are weakest. Identify when it is that you reach for junk or sugar and have a strategy in place to deal with it: eat something healthy before you usually have your urge for something sweet and stave off the hunger pangs before they arise.

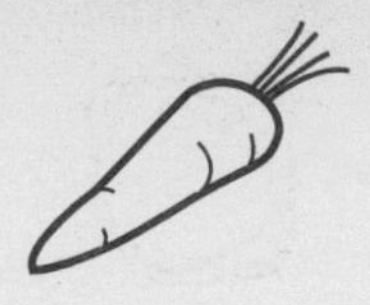

Afternoons are my worst times for eating rubbish. Everyone else goes to the shop for snacks – how can I stop?

Avoid energy dips which is the main reason why you need to snack in the afternoon. Have loads of snacks in your drawer or locker. In summer fresh fruit (strawberries and cherries are a real treat and you can eat lots of them). In winter have a steaming cup of vegetable bouillon, which is just like a broth soup. Have rice crackers, Ryvita and dried apricots, sultanas and bananas handy.

If you have an office, close your office door, or turn away from the chocolate munchers.

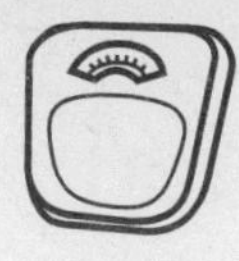

How do you think about your weight?

Getting your mind straight about your body is key. What do we do whenever we lose something? Try and find it again. Let's not focus on 'losing' but on 'getting'. Don't think about losing weight but about getting the body and healthy lifestyle that you want.

My treat is to eat – what'll I do if I have to stop ?

Think of other ways to reward yourself – flowers, a new lip gloss, a new book or CD or flirting with someone you've fancied for ages.

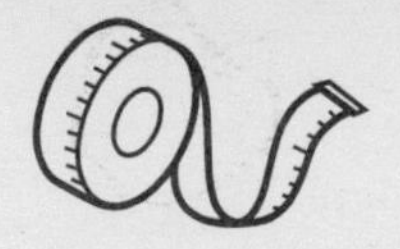

Whenever you feel like you're missing out on food remind yourself of what you'll get in return:

- a hot, slim body
- a great shape in jeans
- more choice in clothes
- you'll be healthier and less likely to have heart disease in later life

Girly don't go there

- milkshake meal substitutes
- jaw wiring
- stomach stapling
- liposuction

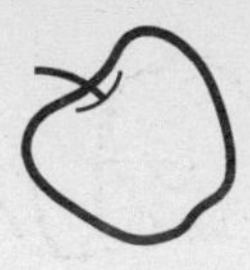

My family are always filling up my plate with seconds and ignore my diet . . .

If you are overweight and need to refuse seconds, then just leave the table as soon as you've had your first plate of food. Take your plate off the table and start the washing up or go to the loo.

They might not be doing it deliberately, it might just be their way of showing their love for you, but don't let them sabotage your careful eating if you really do need to lose weight.

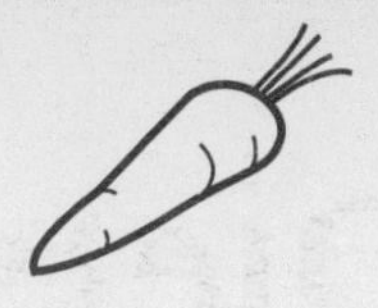

I can't face giving up food, I've done it before and it is always so depressing ...

- Stay away from sad diet foods, thin soups, slimming drinks, too many dry crackers and cold, raw salads. Take more time over preparing your food.

- A salad can be much more delicious if you take the leaves out of the fridge in advance so that they aren't cold and tasteless. Dry roast half-a-dozen pine nuts for a few minutes in a pan; you don't need oil, just toss them frequently so that they roast evenly, and keeping a close watch so that they don't burn – added to your salad they will give a rich, nutty flavour. Then cook a skinless chicken breast and slice it across the breast – you'll have enough for two salads and it will transform the flavour of a boring salad.

Diets

If you are going to go on a diet, choose one that is right for you and your lifestyle – that way you are more likely to stick to it.

Despite the fancy or sometimes downright strange diets that are around, the philosophy behind most diets – even if it is not stated – is to eat fewer calories than the body needs. Then they suggest a maintenance diet once you have reached your ideal weight where your calorie intake should match your energy requirements and in theory you should stay the same weight.

Start by thinking about how much weight you would like to lose. (Remember that a sensible weight loss is 2 lb a week; any more than that and your bone mass starts to decrease, which increases your risk of osteoporosis.)

Think fewer calories – which you will achieve by giving up bad carbs and foods saturated in fat. Exercise 20 minutes per day and you are there.

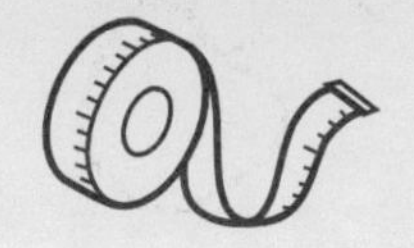

Dr Atkins

The diet:

Cutting out the carbs almost completely: as little as 20 grams at the beginning of the diet. And instead, eat as much protein as you like. Your breakfast can include eggs, bacon, even black pudding if it's your thing.

Even seemingly harmless veg like baked potato (how many times have you eaten them when you've been on a diet? Most of us do!) and sweet potato are out on this diet, as they are high in carbohydrates.

The philosophy is to eat without feeling guilty and still lose weight. This diet not only allows, but positively encourages you, to eat all of the foods that are banned on most other diets.

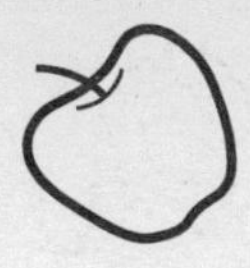

The verdict:

Massively controversial, with many vocal admirers and detractors. *The Sun* is for it; *The Mail* against it.

Renée Zellweger does it, Jennifer Aniston, Minnie Driver and Geri, all noticeably slim, are also devotees. The buxom Nigella Lawson calls it 'the perfect diet for those who love food'. Comic David Baddiel loves it too though Oprah Winfrey claims it didn't do it for her.

Top Atkins tip:

'Cooking your pasta *al dente* (slightly firm to the tooth rather than floppy and overcooked) significantly lowers its glycaemic effects.' In short, there is less of an effect on your blood sugar levels if you cook your pasta a few minutes less. (*Dr Atkins New Diet Revolution*, page 79.)

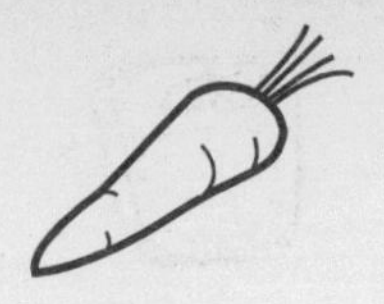

Cabbage soup diet

What is it?

A 7-day cabbage soup diet which also includes specific other vegetables and fruit.

It sounds revolting and is based on a dodgy principle that cabbage has fat-burning properties. Having said that, lots of people claim it works, probably because eating clear soup and lots of fruit and vegetables is similar to a detox diet. And it is bound to be low in calories too.

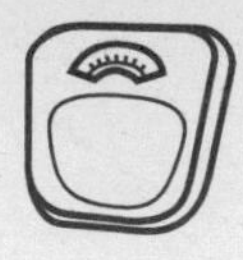

The verdict:

It's a temporary diet, not an eating plan or a food lifestyle that will help you to lose weight permanently. Probably much of the weight loss is fluid.

A nice little mini detox, which will probably help if you want to lose weight quickly to fit into a dress or before you go on holiday. If you want to keep the weight off you'll need to think of a more long-term plan for eating.

You'll find the diet free on the Internet on a number of dieting sites: use a search engine such as Google or Yahoo and type in Cabbage Soup Diet.

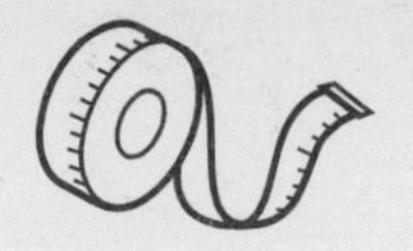

Mind over cream bun

Try the giving-up-smoking techniques. It's not that you can't have chocolate, you can eat the whole bar right now if you want.

If you don't eat the chocolate it's because you've chosen not to have it. Right?!

Isn't there ever a time when a crash diet is ok?

Forget crash diets and quick weight loss unless you've got a GOOD excuse:

Competing in the Miss World pageant; getting married and the dress no longer fits; going to a school or college reunion and an ex you never really got over will be there.

Or an interview for a top job for which you'll need to appear on the ball and hungry, and plump doesn't make the right impression.

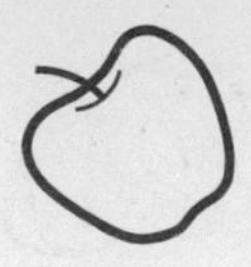

The Fat Flush Plan

The promise: You are only 14 days away from a firmer, leaner body. This diet will help you burn fat faster, detox your system, increase your energy levels and keep your metabolism high.

The author claims that the main problem for overweight people is an overloaded and toxic liver which prevents you from burning fat properly. So part of the fat flush plan is liver detoxification.

Drink eight glasses of cranberry water per day as a fat-flushing food: 1 part cranberry to 4 parts water. (It probably flushes your system in just the same way water does.)

The verdict: I don't recall a single scientific study showing that there is such a thing as fat-burning or fat-flushing foods.
Kate Winslet is said to be a fan, along with Halle Berry and Jennifer Aniston (but which diet isn't she said to be on? I hope Brad appreciates it . . .)

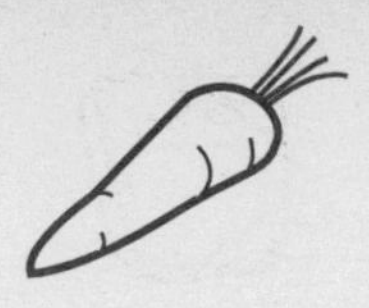

Low-fat diets seem to be unpopular now that Atkins is 'the' diet ...

Low-fat diets avoid all foods which are high in fats. They recommend removing all fat from meat and the skin from chicken. Plus they advise cutting down on, or cutting out, butter and dairy products.

You need to be careful of prepackaged low-fat foods such as yoghurt and biscuits, as they are often higher in sugar as, without the fat, the food has less taste.

There is a temptation on a low-fat diet to fill up on carbs but this will undo any good you have done by cutting out fats.

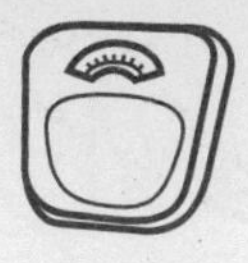

There is a wide acceptance now that good fats are necessary for us to be healthy. So keep on cutting the fat from meat if you prefer it that way but make sure you have oils such as olive oil and at least some dairy products. Margarine, and foods that contain fats and carbs such as pastries, donuts and croissants, should be cut out altogether.

You must also have oily fish or if you don't like fish then find yourself a good supplement from your health food store.

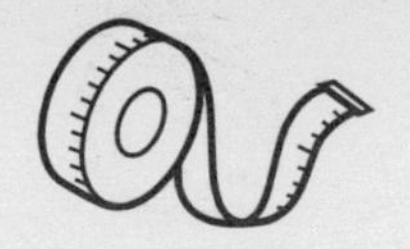

But which diet really works?

And after all of that information consider this: findings from a recent scientific study showed that on the Atkins diet (giving up bread, pasta and rice), you lose weight faster than on a low-fat diet but that after 12 months the weight loss is the same.

So both low-carb and low-fat diets work: Atkins is faster but for the long term either will help you to lose weight.

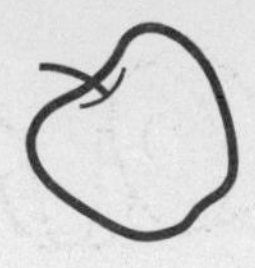

Calorie-free foods

The good news is that some food is free food: okay, the bad news is that they're not that exciting but you can have as much as you want. Pickles, cucumber, herbal tea, salad and veg (potato, sweetcorn and sweet potato excluded).

You can make a really cool Greek dip, tzatziki, with cucumber, low-fat yoghurt and garlic. Shred the veg and stir into the yoghurt.

Those little baby gherkins (cornichons) are really tasty and crunchy and are great with drinks. You can eat as much as you want…

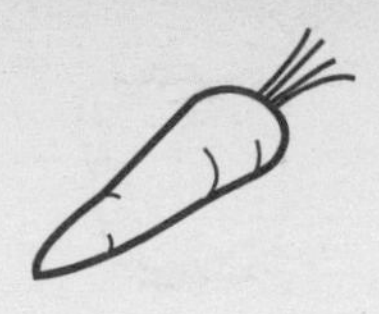

Yuk, low-carb diets are revolting. I hate fat and always avoid it ...

Don't worry if low-carb diets don't appeal to you. They're not for everybody.

If you don't like fatty food and tend to not eat much protein you need to be careful that you are not filling up on bread, pasta and rice. Anyone who wants to lose weight should reduce the amount of carbs they eat and to replace them you'll probably need to eat more protein. It needn't be steaks and bacon butties if you don't fancy that kind of food. Chicken, fish, eggs, all are full of protein and it doesn't have to be grilled chicken with one lettuce leaf either. There are all sorts of things you can eat. Look for a good cook-book to give you some ideas.

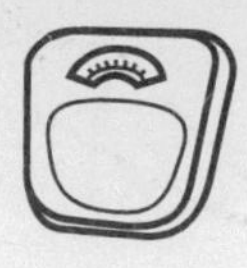

You need fats in your diet to stay healthy and to provide your body with essential fatty acids: dairy, meat, fish, olive oil, avocados, rapeseed oil, flaxseed oil, pumpkin seeds. Consider taking a good supplement if you know you don't get many fats in your diet: ask at your health store.

Keep these fats in your diet: they're healthy and essential for good skin, help ward off depression.

At least 25 per cent of your diet should be made up of good fats.

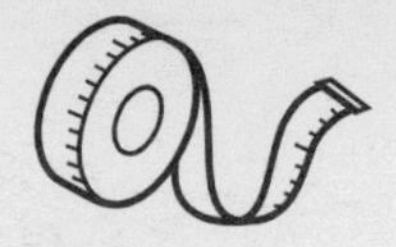

Forget it!

Any diet which gives you Ryvita for lunch (fine as a snack but they're not a meal) or overly restricting portions, telling you that you can only have 6 grapes with your lunch. How depressing!

Illegal foods:

- fizzy drinks
- pasta or rice more than once a week
- crisps
- sweets
- cake
- chips more than once a week
- croissant or pastry more than once a week

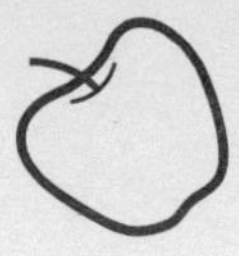

Skinny girls are so annoying! What do they eat?

- They deliberately eat chocolate in front of you to give the impression they can eat all they like, and then probably don't eat any more all week.
- They bang on about how much they ate at the weekend.
- They sigh over how 'fat' they are … when they are a teeny bit premenstrually bloated.
- They pick at their food, when they look like they really need a good meal.

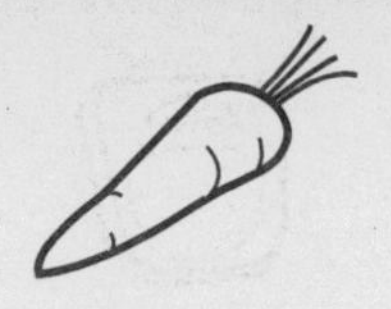

Bingeing

Can happen occasionally and usually makes you feel dreadful afterwards. Forget it, move on, but do get some help if it becomes a regular thing or if it is more serious than eating a whole packet of biscuits.

Geri Halliwell has recounted fishing a cake out of a rubbish bin and eating the whole thing. Not healthy!

If you are making yourself sick after a binge, talk to your doctor about it right away.

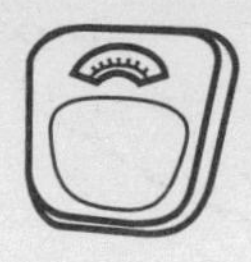

I want to lose weight fast: what is a realistic amount to lose?

1 to 2 lbs a week is safe and realistic – any more than that and you'll probably feel awful, may be risking your health, plus you'll probably put the weight back on again anyway once you stop your crash diet.

If you really must go on a crash diet then have a sensible eating plan ready so that when you come off the diet, you can eat properly to maintain the weight you're at, and keep off the weight you have lost.

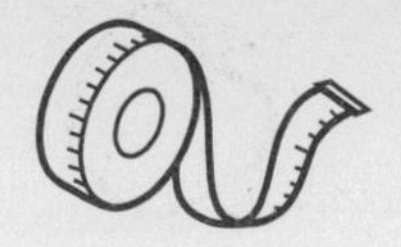

Weighing in

Don't become obsessed with the scales – daily weighing is not going to help. Weigh yourself no more than once a month and use a better, more relevant measure of success, like how you look in the mirror. And nominate a close-fitting dress that is your measure of weight going up and down. A bit snug is fine – you'll have monthly hormonal variations. Straining at the seams and maybe you're going in too hard with the chocolate and lager.

If you don't believe this try it out for yourself. Eat as you usually would and weigh yourself morning and night for a week. The variations may bear no relation to what you're actually eating.

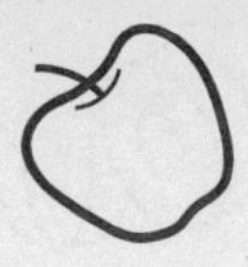

Surely a can of fizzy drink can't do me any harm ...

Fizzy drinks are a complete waste of calories and they're bad for you in every way. Used sparingly, Coke for a hangover gives you a sugar rush and temporarily makes you feel better, but it will make you reach for more sugary food once your blood sugar dips again.

Plus, it's a hip-bulging drink if you drink it regularly. And it doesn't fill you up but you get a huge whack of calories .

Calorie count: 135 calories in a can of Coke, 80 in lemonade.

Have a can of Coke every day, plus an extra can on Saturday morning to sort out your hangover, that's 1080 calories per week. If you're dieting, trying to stick to 1200 cals a day, then your week's Coke intake is close to a whole day's food intake!

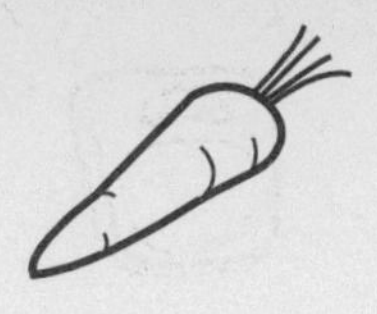

The Zone Diet

The diet:
The main principle of the Zone diet is that you eat foods in the following percentages:
40% carbs
30% protein
30% fat

The verdict: It's complicated and despite all its fanciness it essentially comes down to being a low-calorie diet of about 800–1200 cals per day.

The Zone diet allows you more carbs than the Atkins diet but is a bit tricky. It requires you to eat six times a day – okay if you're not busy, but who isn't . . .

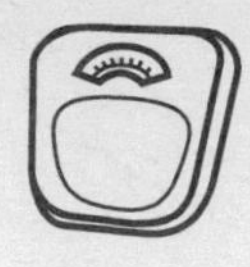

The bonus: You don't have to do any exercise on the Zone diet. It is nutritionally sound and balanced and you may lose weight as you'll be eating fewer calories. There's no guarantee you'd keep the weight off though without exercise.

Sandra Bullock is said to be a Zone fan.

Being thin isn't a magical solution.
'I thought that being thinner would solve all of my problems and make me really happy. I love the way I look but the problems didn't vanish with the weight ...'

Anonymous

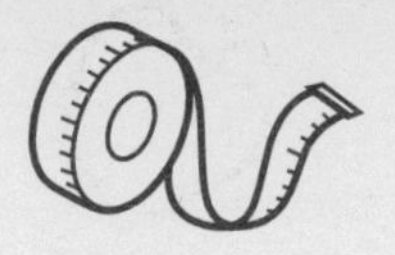

I'm confused – do carbs make you fat, or foods that are high in fat such as meat and dairy foods?

For a long time there was an assumption that fat made us fat. It now appears that certain fats are vital to our good health and will not make us put on weight if we eat the right fats in moderation.

The problem with carbs (pasta, bread, rice) is that when you eat them they send blood sugar levels soaring and you just want to eat more and more. Whereas fat (dairy, meat, oils, nuts and seeds) fills you up and leaves you with a more satisfied feeling for longer, and they don't make you crave more.

Avoid fats such as margarine or anything containing hydrogenated fats: check the label of your peanut butter and buy one that doesn't contain these fats, from your health food store.

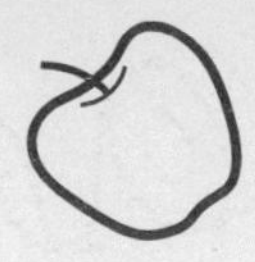

Avocados …

… are high in fat but it is good, healthy fat that gives you a full and satisfied feeling. And because they are creamy in texture you feel you are treating yourself.

Carbs are my weakness – I adore them …

Have some carbs if you really feel you need them, just not at every meal. And go for the more complex carbs (which don't affect your blood sugar level as badly). Cut pasta down to once a week. Have baked beans on toast, rice (brown instead of white), dried apricots, wholewheat bread.

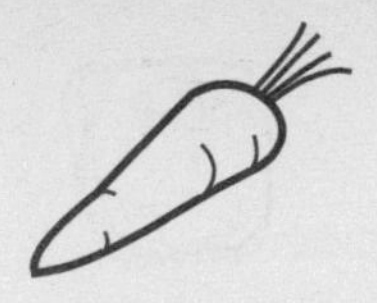

How can I make this whole weight-loss thing less painful? I hate giving up food ...

Harmless things to give up:

- sugar in your tea and coffee (1 teaspoon = 20 calories)
- sugar on cereal (20–35 calories)
- beer – have wine instead
- crisps – have crudités
- butter for frying – use olive oil
- butter on your bread
- fried bacon – have grilled instead
- fried eggs – have them scrambled
- sugar puffs – have muesli
- Diet Coke – have apple juice

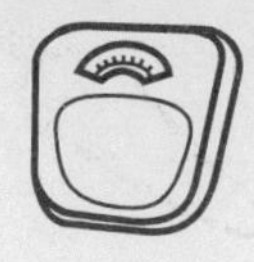

Skinny girls do

- drink v&t instead of lager
- dash around instead of moving slowly

Skinny girls don't

- always choose the choc pud
- have crisps every lunchtime with their sarnie

Snack time

- kitchen timer for when you're at home
- at work – alarm on your computer
- or alarm on watch or mobile

Set the alarm and then don't think about it – you'll get a pleasant surprise when the alarm goes off

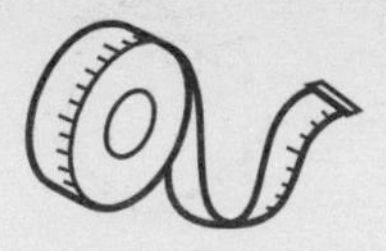

10 reasons not to be skinny

- wrinkles will show up on your face
- you'll look older
- people think you're anorexic if you don't eat
- people think you're bulimic if you're skinny and you eat a lot
- your boobs will shrink
- a curvier body looks better naked
- there'd be nothing for your man to hang on to
- you'll feel the cold more
- people tell you you're skinny all the time

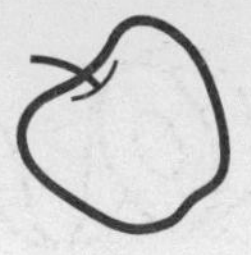

Classic excuses for being fat

- big bones
- slow metabolism
- women need chocolate
- women's bodies are programmed to make fat (this is true but you can still do something about it) – they make fat more easily and release it more slowly than men do

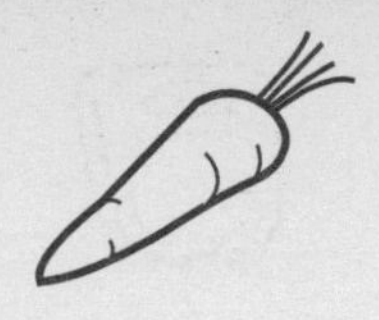

100-calorie snacks

- 2 squares Dairy Milk chocolate
- 2 oatcakes
- any piece of fruit
- small pot of low-fat yoghurt and a banana
- a palmful of sunflower and pumpkin seeds
- 20 almonds
- 8 dried apricots

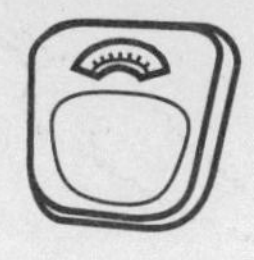

I can't stop thinking about food – I'm obsessed.

Did you see those 'celebs' on *I'm a Celebrity, Get Me Out of Here?* They're not starving yet all they can think about is food and that's because the food available to them is restricted. They perform all manner of hideous tasks with rats and maggots to earn food. Then they storm the camera room, threatening a mutiny if they don't get more food to eat.

The point is, if you're going without food then your blood sugar levels will drop, you'll feel weak and irritable and food will be all you can think about.

Don't let yourself get to this point. Feed yourself properly so you're not feeling deprived.

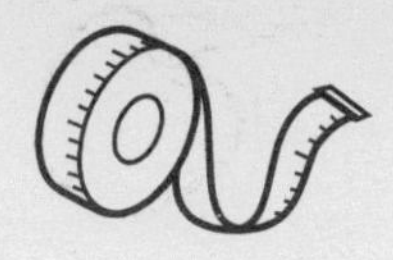

Celeb diets

For celebs their bodies are their main work tool. Their job depends on them looking their best so they'll go to extreme lengths for the sake of their appearance.

It isn't really necessary for us mere mortals to go to such extremes to look good. And probably not possible either … At their disposal they have a team of helpers: celebrity chefs, personal trainers and dieticians, as well as unlimited funds to buy the best food available.

They work out hard to get in shape for their films but then it often falls apart in between. Think of Russell-5-chins-Crowe who managed to hunk up superbly for *Gladiator*. Whenever the paparazzi snap him off duty he always looks a couple of stone overweight.

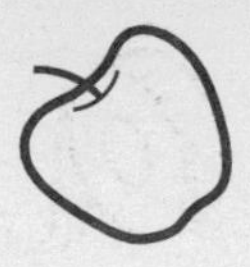

I'm not really fat, I'm preparing for my latest role …

Much more convincing than Winona Ryder's claims that she shoplifted only to prepare for a new film, Renée Zellweger genuinely did become porky just for the sake of her art. She gained 2 stone for her film role as Bridget Jones.

How did she do it? She included loads of Big Macs, donuts, crisps, pizza and pasta into her daily diet. Feel worried, very worried if this sounds like your regular diet. It's really simple to see how this leads to an extra 2 stone in weight.

Did you notice, though, that when she ran through the streets as Bridget Jones, after her man, wearing only her big pants and a sweater, that nothing wobbled as she ran? A body stocking perhaps? Or was she big but fit from exercising?

Then there is Tom Hanks who lost 55 lb for his *Castaway* role by eating only coffee and apples. Not an appealing thought.

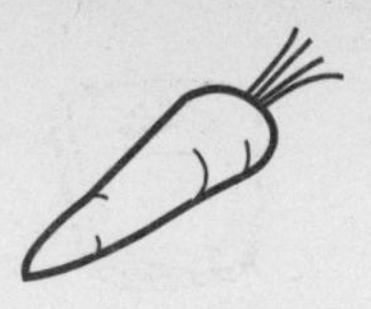

It's never too late to change your body …

… as Demi Moore has shown, getting into shape – serious shape – after three kids and aged 42 for the film, *Charlie's Angels* 2.

Ashtanga Yoga has surely helped, but her diet *is* a little odd. Under the guidance of a top restaurateur and chef to the stars, she mainly eats raw foods, but chomps her way through cakes, pies and puddings too.

Sounds good? Hang on a minute, though – the cakes were made of pumpkin and carob seeds, the pies made of … do you really want me to go on?

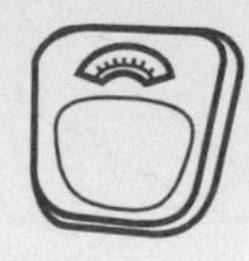

Accept your weight

- We're a celeb-obsessed nation and we love to watch them and copy them. If there's a particular celeb whose body you'd love to have, have another look – do they seem healthy and happy? Or do they have a pale, pinched-looking face?

- If they look gorgeous, healthy and cheerful, then find out what their exercise programme is and follow it.

- The downside – even celebs can't buy a hot-looking body, it does involve work, and you'll find out first-hand what it costs them in working to get and keep that body.

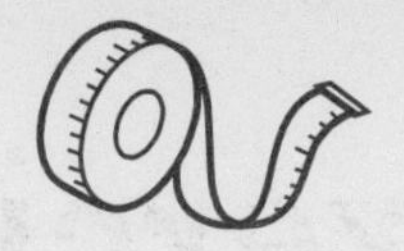

Will a detox diet help me to lose weight?

The main way in which a detox diet works is that you avoid salt, which will help banish water retention, and you also take in fewer calories, as the basis of most detox diets is fruit and veg.

You will lose weight on a detox diet – you'll find that the first phase of weight loss will be a loss of excess fluid.

Celebs such as Madonna, Kylie, Kate Moss, Elle Macpherson and Liz Hurley swear by a detox now and then.

Most pharmacies do a detox kit to help you but a cheap, simple and not overly taxing detox is the Cabbage Soup Diet, see page 86.

Exercise

You will have to do some and that's the truth.

If you're serious about losing weight, how hard can a 15–20 mins brisk walk 3 or 4 times a week be?

Do it at lunchtime and set yourself a destination, with a treat at the end of it:

- Monday – the newsagents to buy a glossy magazine
- Tuesday – a cappuccino from your fave café
- Wednesday – some new make-up
- Thursday – a smoothie or a freshly squeezed juice
- Friday – a cake, hurrah!

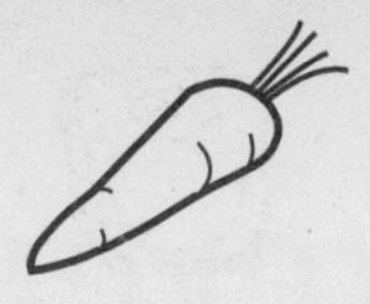

I never have any time for exercise, what can I do?

Oh, and you don't have time to go to Top Shop or Next either do you? And you know all that stuff about getting off the bus/train one stop earlier and walking, taking the stairs rather than the lift – bored? Heard it before? Yeah, well do it and stop moaning.

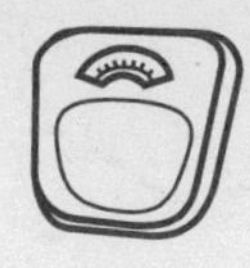

Assess your level of activity

If you are 9 stone and pretty active and then your life changes, so that the amount you exercise or are active decreases, this may mean that your daily need for calories drops by as much as 400–500 calories. In other words you can't carry on eating the same amount of food and expect not to gain weight. Every time you make a change in lifestyle reassess the amount and type of food you eat.

Has your lifestyle changed recently? If it has, or if you know that it is going to change, prepare for it by altering how many calories you eat.

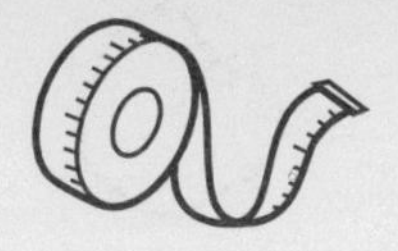

Answer these questions:

- Have you stopped walking part way to work and started driving?
- Got a new boyfriend and you don't go out clubbing – and dancing – any more?
- Has your toddler gone to school and you're doing much less running around after her?
- Have you been promoted from the shop-floor to an office job?
- Are you in a new job where you don't get a chance to go for a walk at lunchtime?

If you've answered yes to any of these questions then you'll need to reconsider how much you eat. Your energy requirements will be fewer than when you were more active, so if you continue to eat in the same way as you have been, you'll put on weight.

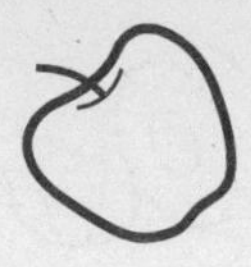

If I exercise can I eat anything I want and not put on weight?

You can't exercise away an unhealthy sugar and fat-laden diet. You'll probably find that without a reduced intake of calories, if you eat lots of food, and that food is high in sugar and fat, exercise won't make any difference to your weight. You'll firm up the bulk you have so you'll have firm thighs but big ones …

So, sorry, while exercise shapes your body you'll also need to eat sensibly if you want to lose weight.

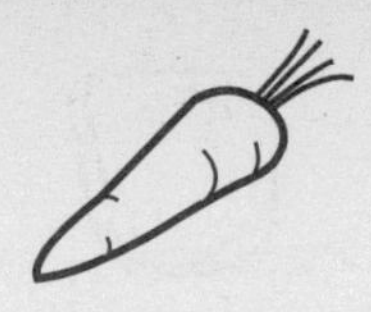

My waist is fine but my bottom needs work – what can I do?

Dieting won't get to your problem areas; in fact you lose weight off your belly first which will only make your bum look bigger. You'll need to either accept that that is how you are built or reduce your calorie intake and target your rear with exercise. Firm it up, Kylie-stylie.

If it's any comfort even skinny girls can have wobbly bums and cellulite; the fact is that most bums need exercise to look good.

Especially beyond a certain age.

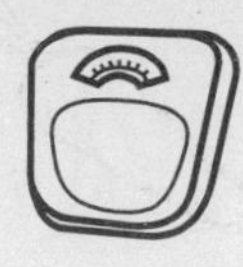

Good exercises for your bottom include:

- buttocks clenches wherever you can – they're much easier to do undetected when you're wearing a skirt or have a coat on
- leg raises: get down on all fours and keeping your leg bent push your leg out behind you. You can do this watching the telly or put a magazine on the floor in front of you
- swimming: breaststroke especially is good for your bottom; sidestroke will work your inner thighs. You'll see noticeable results in just 2 weeks if you swim 3 or more times a week

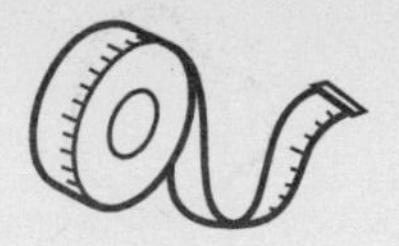

I've got the biggest bum in the whole world ...

You wouldn't be exaggerating just a little bit, would you? Lucky you if you do have a sizeable bottom – half the female population are desperate for a shapely bum like J-Lo's.

Get it into shape, firm it up, shop for a good pair of well-fitting, flattering trousers and enjoy the attention.

If you are carrying extra weight, a healthy-sized ass is the best place to have it: it poses no threat to your health as it is where women are biologically programmed to store fat.

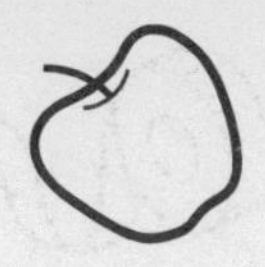

You can't choose where to lose weight but you can target the trouble spot with exercise to improve its appearance. When you lose weight bear in mind that you lose it in this order:

- stomach/belly area
- face
- between your shoulder blades
- hips and thighs

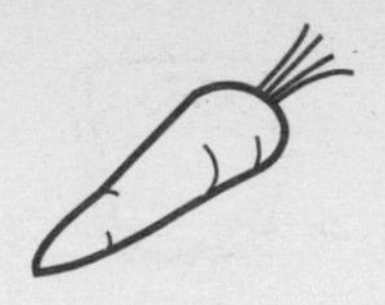

What can I do to get the body shape I want?

The body shape you have and where you tend to lay down fat is something you inherit, sadly, so you can't make total changes. Some people are prone to putting on weight on their tummy first, some people on their hips and bums. You could say that J-Lo has a big bum – well, she has – but what she also has is a tight and toned big bum which is why it looks so good. Work to tighten up and streamline what you've got is the moral of this story.

Exercise – take it where you can.
It doesn't have to be the same kind of exercise every day – you don't have to commit to a weekly gym or aerobics session. Clubbing, shopping, running for the bus, and sex, all count as exercise.

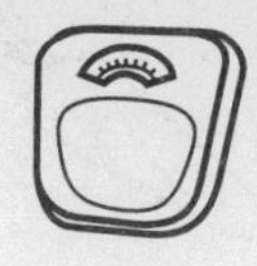

Are you sure – do I really have to exercise?

There's convincing evidence that it is a lack of exercise that is making us fat. Our calorific intake as a whole in the UK has fallen. So we eat less – yet we're getting fatter? How can that be? We sit in bars, we watch loads of TV, many of us work in jobs where we sit for most of the day.

Sorry, but you've got to get moving to lose weight.

The plateau

Exercise helps to reduce that maddening plateau effect where you stop losing weight after an initial good burst of weight loss.

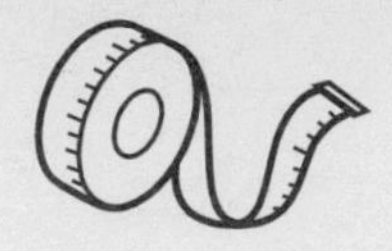

I've joined a gym loads of times but I always drop out …

You're not alone if that makes you feel any better: over 60 per cent of people who join a gym in the New Year will have dropped out six months later. If you really can't stick to the gym or an exercise routine then save your pennies (by not joining the gym) and get yourself a personal trainer. If you can't afford a trainer then get an exercise buddy and motivate each other to keep going.

Maybe signing up for classes rather than the gym would suit you. They're fun and can be more sociable, and if you choose the right class you'll get some seriously groovy music to exercise to.

For the desperately hard-to-get-moving: make sure your gym has a TV and do your workout so that your time on the exercise bike coincides with EastEnders.

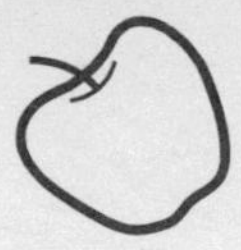

Telly chubbies

Don't despair – there are loads of exercises you can do in front of the box:

- leg raises
- buttock clenches
- skipping
- bouncing on a mini trampoline
- clenching pillows – or a man or a bag of sweets – between your thighs (Note: eating the sweets after you've finished exercising with them would probably cancel out the effects of the exercise, tee hee!)
- stepping up and down on a small step-ladder

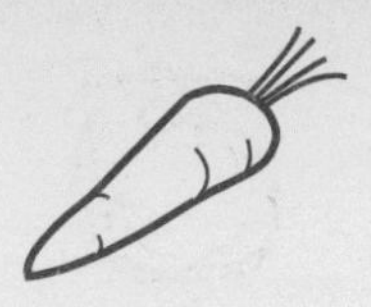

Help, it's so long since I've exercised, the last time I did any I was wearing a gym kit at school ...

- Start gradually, 10 minutes at first is fine, with some gentle exercise such as walking, cycling or swimming.
- Increase the time and vigorousness of the exercise when you feel more confident.
- Kid yourself you're just catching up on office gossip: go for a walk with the girls at lunchtime.
- Set a goal, go to a bar or restaurant you'd usually drive to and walk it instead.

If you're very overweight and unfit consult your doctor before doing anything more energetic than walking.

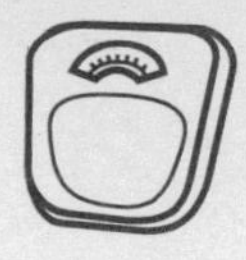

Focus on your body in a positive way.

- You're not allowed to eat rubbish food but you are allowed to have fab massages.

- Get yourself some stickers and put one in a book every time you would have bought a chocolate bar but stopped yourself. Add up the figures at the end of the month – you can probably afford a massage to get your circulation going and help with your weight loss.

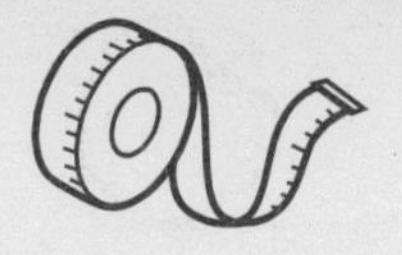

The apple and the pear, the good news and the bad news.

For **apple** shapes (carrying weight around the waist), the good news is that fat above the hips is the easiest to shift; fat below the hips is much harder to shed.

For **pear** shapes (carrying weight on the hips and bottom), although it might be harder to shift fat from the bottom – probably because we are built for fat storage there – fat below the hips carries a much smaller threat to health than above, so pear shapes don't really need to get rid of it. You can keep your J-Lo bum without harming your health.

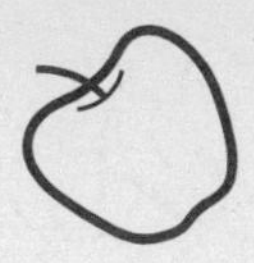

Help, I've got an unattractive Michelin-man tyre around my waist.

It must go! Carrying excess fat around your waist is a clue that your body might be having trouble dealing with the sugar you put into it. I don't just mean sweets and cakes but carbohydrates such as white bread, pasta and rice. (Any low-carb diet will give you a fuller list of the foods that are high in carbs, or check the Internet.)

Luckily for you the waist is one of the first places you lose weight.

That's a good incentive to do something about it, as you can get results really quickly.

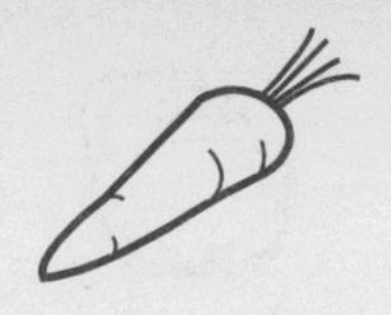

Fast food dance

The good news: You can dance to burn off your fast food.

- A burger and fries will take 2 hours, 10 minutes
- Fish and chips, 1 hour, 25 minutes

The bad news: It's still junk so don't have it too often.

What's the point of exercise? I don't want to end up all muscly …

People who don't take any exercise eat more than those who do. If you exercise for just half an hour a day you'll be less likely to overeat.

If you eat because you're depressed or lonely, exercise can help. Exercise makes you feel better. It makes you feel more optimistic about life, the universe, everything. Try skipping – it will remind you of happy days as a kid, tra-la-la-la.

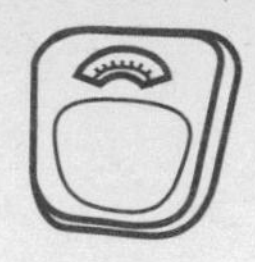

After a session at the gym I'm so hungry that I blow it by grabbing a take-away on the way home.

Keep a snack in your gym bag to eat after your workout. Eating after exercise will boost your energy levels, which in turn will stop your metabolism from slowing down. The longer you keep your metabolism functioning at a high rate the more calories you will burn up.

Girly donut exercises

If you really want it here's what you have to do to earn it:
20 minutes of aerobics, swimming or jogging, or 25 minutes of dancing ...

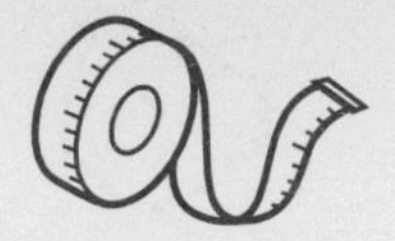

I hate the gym and I feel like a prat jogging around the streets.

Try these 'they're so much fun I can't believe they're exercise' suggestions! (Sooorry ...!)

- bouncing on the bed – it's not just for kids
- space hoppers – take one to the park
- frisbee – on the beach, in the park
- a brisk walk to the pub
- sex (again ...)
- trying on clothes and rushing from shop to shop
- rowing a boat – on water, or on the rowing machine
- skating – ice, roller, blades
- DIY – holding the ladder counts too
- clubbing – dancing or posing
- DIY fake tanning – it takes a lot of effort to reach every bit of your body

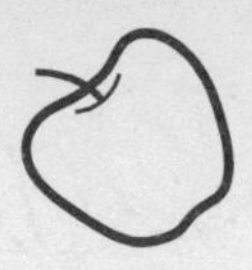

A happy thought:

You can achieve twice as much in half the time when you exercise in water, whether it be an exercise class, or just treading water, or hanging on to the side of the pool and doing leg raises. The resistance of the water means that the exercise is much more effective.

Comforting girly thoughts

If you do just 5 mins exercise per day more than you do now you'll be well on your way to weight loss.

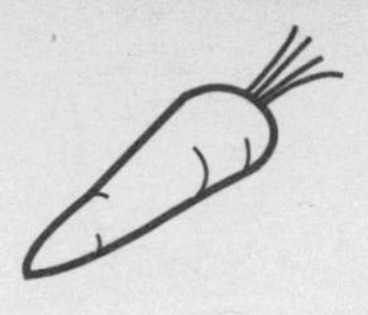

How do I choose the right exercise for me?

Exercise classes go in and out of fashion: one day it's hot, the next day it's not. There are so many classes you can take: from step to kick-boxing and Pilates.

Yoga has been the uber-trendy class for ages. It's thanks to Madonna, Gwyneth and other high-profile devotees – that most of us have a yoga mat lurking in the back of our cupboards.

Loads of people rave about yoga but if you found it too boring to exercise without music, never fear – aerobics is back in vogue.

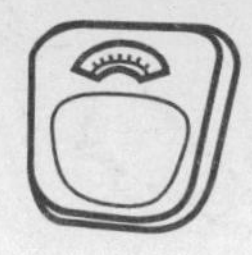

Aerobics

Aerobics is retro-cool, it works, done with weights it sorts out your body to keep your heart and lungs working as they should, and it also helps ward off osteoporosis. And it's back in a big way – ask your mum if she still has her Jane Fonda workout video, find one in a charity shop or find a class to attend and get going.

And, just one session of aerobic exercise can help reduce anxiety for anything up to six hours.

Tai chi

Tai chi improves your posture and gives you a stronger, leaner body. If you practise it a couple of times a week it will help to tone your muscles, boost your circulation and is a really good choice if you can't take strenuous exercise for any reason. Great if you have a bad back or if you're pregnant.

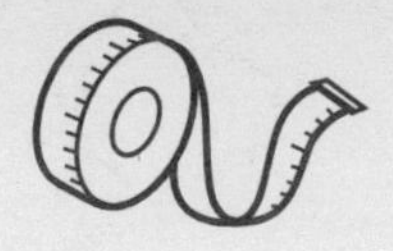

Swimming

Backstroke is the best stroke: it burns off calories faster than any other style of swimming. You can see the results in two weeks of swimming twice a week.

Pilates

Pilates improves posture and flexibility. It strengthens your joints and will make you generally stronger all over. It will also improve your appearance as it will make you look taller.

Yoga

Yoga tones your body and increases your suppleness and flexibility. It strengthens your muscles and improves the functioning of your internal organs. You will see results after a month or so of weekly classes.

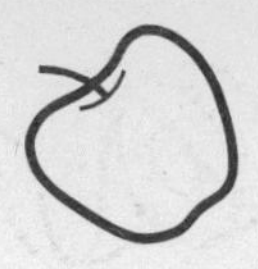

Running

Running is free, and easy to do any time. You'll need good trainers to prevent jarring of joints and spine. If you feel any discomfort then stop and walk until you feel better.

Tell me again why I need to exercise, I'm not convinced ...

Exercise kick-starts your metabolism, firms your body and makes you feel good (once you've done it).

Your other option is to stay on a diet for life, constantly worrying about your weight, wishing you were slimmer ... not a very pretty thought ...

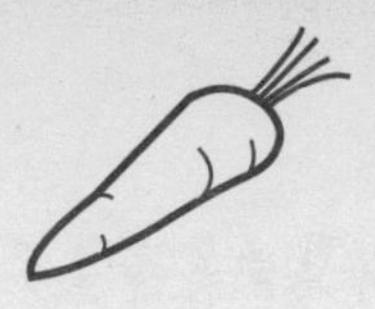

Smug girly

Taking exercise can boost your metabolism for up to 24 hours after you finish exercising, meaning you'll burn calories faster, even when you're resting.

Jog or walk briskly to your mate's house for a girls' night in and you can feel secretly smug, because not only will you have exercised but you'll also still be burning off calories faster than your mates when you're sitting relaxing on the sofa, drinking wine.

Staying In

(Entertaining)

When I'm trying to diet all I can think about is food and – well, I become obsessed. Help!

- Surround yourself with food! Yes, you heard right.
- The biggest mistake you can make is to clear out your fridge and cupboards replacing the food with only low-fat stuff and Ryvita crackers; and then avoid going out to dinner and generally deprive yourself of food.
- Make your food list of all the foods that you can and will eat. You can have an everyday list – the stuff that's healthy and will fill you up without making you fat; a once-a-week list –

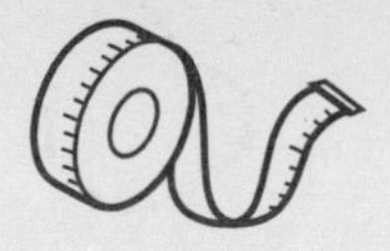

croissants are on mine; and a once-a-month list – a jam donut for me.

- Get out all your favourite cookbooks, or get a new one if all of yours are cake-baking books. Make long lists of healthy meals and shop for the ingredients. Spend an entire day preparing, cooking, eating and then inviting your mates round to eat lots of gorgeous (healthy) wonderful food.

- Try to have your cupboards stocked with good ingredients and your fridge full of healthy, fresh food. This is easier to do if you live with others and they want to eat well too; tough if you live with junk fiends, and also hard if you live on your own (see page 158 for how to get around this).

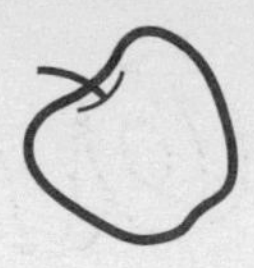

- **Always** have chocolate in the house. Treat yourself to an expensive box of chocolates or a bar of some fab rich, dark chocolate, and allow yourself two pieces after dinner each night. You'll look forward to it and feel incredibly virtuous at only having eaten two pieces.

- If you binge on it and gobble it all up in one day don't give yourself a hard time about it, you're just not allowed any more until next week. So there!

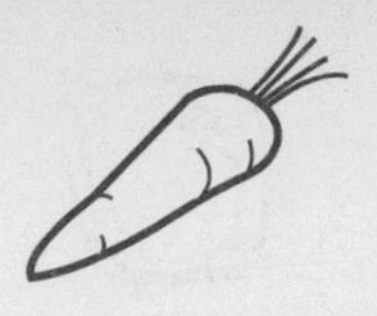

I get really upset at the thought of living on baked potatoes and steamed fish for weeks on end.

You don't need to.

If you're having people over, make an easy low-fat dip with lots of crunchy crudités followed by a healthy home-made burger (no bun), see recipe opposite, some boiled new potatoes, sliced avocado on the side, a tomato salsa and a green leaf salad with tasty dressing. Make a huge batch of burgers and you'll have them ready-made in the freezer for weeks to come, just waiting to be grilled.

Have fruit or a sorbet to follow instead of ice cream or cake.

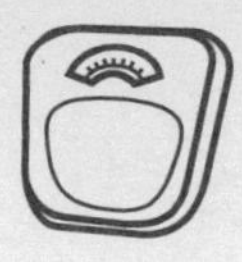

Home-made burgers: So easy. Combine extra-lean mince with chopped parsley and finely chopped onion. Add a little chilli or coriander, or a splash of soy sauce if you want to. (The quantities are up to you, 500g of mince should make about 6–8 good-sized burgers.) Simply shape them and cook them under the grill.

Tomato salsa: Finely chopped tomatoes, chopped onion, coriander. Mix the ingredients together and pour over a little olive oil.

To drink: Make a low-cal punchy drink with white or red wine combined with sparkling mineral water or soda with loads of fruit thrown in. Add a glass of cranberry or orange juice, the no-added-sugar sort.

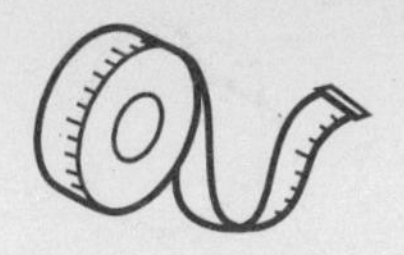

Girly fridge mantras

If you're up for a laugh:

- go ahead be a fat pig
- eat that chocolate, build that arse
- fill on up, Fatso

or if you prefer to be positive and a bit hippy about it:

- I am getting slimmer every day in every way
- each day I find it easier to eat good, healthy food

No kicking the fridge in a fit of temper please.

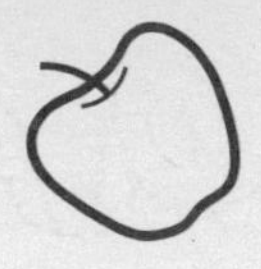

It's so depressing, all of the food you can eat on a diet is horrible ...

You can make your food tastier. Marinating will give your food extra flavour so you get maximum taste. It really sexes up the flavours of simple food.

You can marinate your meat or fish in yoghurt, wine, lemon juice, herbs, spices, freshly ground black pepper – all add flavour. (Not all at once though ...)

A marinade of a teaspoon of honey, dash of soy sauce, grated ginger and a dash of fish sauce gives fab Thai flavours to any meat (marinate for at least 4 hours). Then grill or barbeque the meat. Eat with a tomato and onion salad and some green beans.

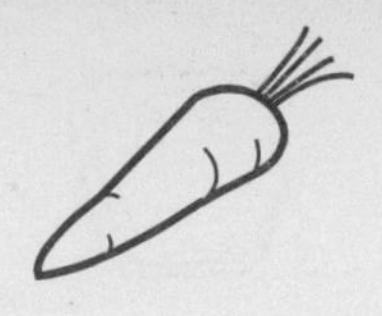

Dieting girly's revenge

On a diet? Don't suffer alone!

Invite your skinny mates round for dinner. Make them a chilli, using extra-lean beef mince with brown rice and topped with low-fat cheese.

Make them unknowingly eat low-fat food at every course, including low-fat wine and finishing with diabetic, sugar-free chocolates. Yum, yum!

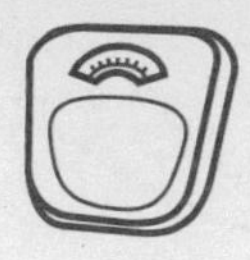

Girly danger times

Often it's when you're at home that you're most at risk of an eating-fest. Boredom, putting off the ironing, watching TV or when you have your period are all testing times when you'll be tempted to eat the wrong things.

Keep your fridge and your cupboards clear of the wrong snack foods. They're too easy to break out and eat.

Make sure you always have healthy snacks, fruit, fresh and dried, seeds and nuts (but not salted peanuts or cashews), plain crackers and rye or wholewheat bread.

Think ahead for main meals so that you don't get overly hungry and eat badly.

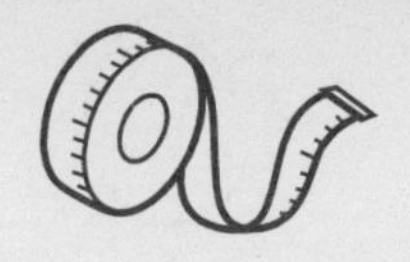

What should I eat for breakfast? I'll really miss my bacon sarnie.

Keep your bacon sarnie, just make sure that you grill, not fry, the bacon and don't overdo the butter on the bread or toast.

We're always nagged to eat a good breakfast but sometimes you might find that if it is too hearty you'll need lunch earlier followed by snacks all afternoon. (Is there any truth to the theory that your stomach gets stretched and expects more, the more it gets?)

Watch how what you eat affects you – if you keep a food diary note down how hungry you feel again after each different breakfast that you have.

What you might also find is that a breakfast of a large chocolate-covered cappuccino and a croissant sets the tone for the day in an entirely different way. You'll probably be starving by 11am and want rubbish food all day.

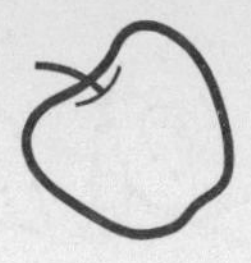

Try and figure out which breakfast has the best effect on you: perhaps porridge or cereal topped with some fruit will satisfy you and keep your blood sugar levels steady.

Water, water everywhere

When you're at home you'll find it easier to drink more water. Drink it instead of fizzy or flavoured drinks and not only will you drop unnecessary calories you'll also flush out toxins and impurities and keep your skin hydrated and looking good.

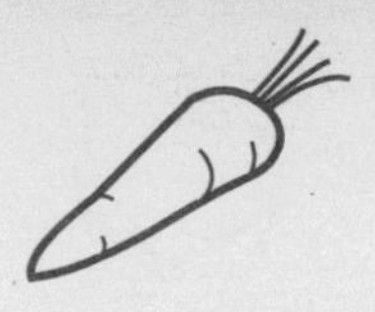

What's lurking in your cupboard?

- Do a spot-check of your cupboards: there is no way that you have Pop-Tarts, Sugar Puffs or CocoPops, is there ...?

- On the inside of the cupboard keep a list of foods that you know you can eat without putting on weight – and there are loads of them.

- Plan your shopping and cooking in advance so you don't resort to eating junk.

- Always read packets before you buy. Avoid sugar: you particularly need to watch out for low-fat products which are often full of sugar to make up for having so little flavour.

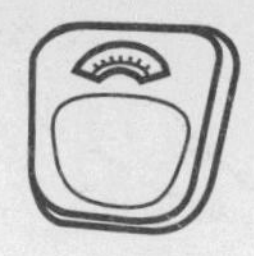

Always buy mini packs if you buy packs of anything for a treat, like dried fruit, crisps or biscuits. If you open a family-size bag it will be that much harder to resist finishing the entire thing.

King- or family-size packs are a marketing ploy to make us think we're getting better value when really all we're getting is fatter …

Your freezer

Always have home-made or shop-bought fresh soups ready to defrost for when you haven't got time to cook.

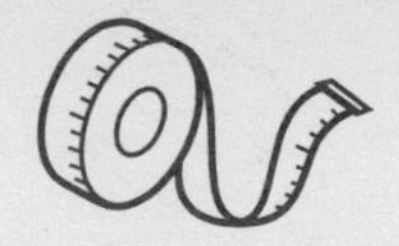

Help - every time I try to eat sensibly I always fail with the same foods that I love.

Find a substitute. For instance if you love ice cream, make some fresh fruit low-fat or full-fat frozen yoghurt ice lollies. Use rich fruit like berries (if you're on the Atkins diet berries are the recommended fruit) and you won't miss the ice cream. Bananas make a more creamy ice lolly recipe.

Girly food trade-off

If you give up sugar in your tea you can have an extra square of chocolate instead. Train yourself out of it, you'll soon get used to doing without it.

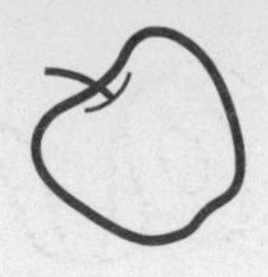

Weakness substitutes

ice cream	yoghurt pops
crisps	blue taco chips if you're in a rush, or crudités with hummus if you're feeling like something crunchy
chocolate	a smaller amount, and you don't need it every day
fried breakfast	the same but grill everything instead
beer	wine instead as it has fewer calories and is lower in carbohydrate, but go easy (as if!) as it has a much higher alcohol content

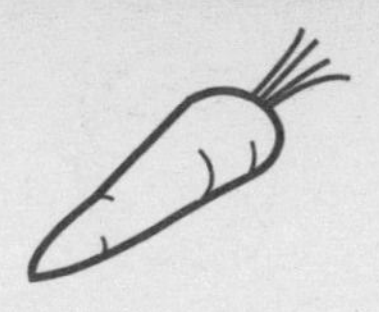

It's all very well to try to eat properly but what about coping with housemates or a junk-addicted family?

It's much easier to eat well if you live with others and they want to eat well too, but tough if you live with junk fiends; in fact you may never get the right eating habits if you smell their takeaways or egg and chips for dinner night after night. Perhaps you need to make the move to living with someone who eats good food.

It can also be hard if you live on your own. Make big batches when you cook and freeze some for later so that you don't need to cook every night. Soups, burgers, fishcakes, stews and curries can all be made in this way. It is especially good in winter to have this kind of comfort food available: if you have a bad day and need to give yourself a lovely meal and a glass of wine you'll have it on hand. If

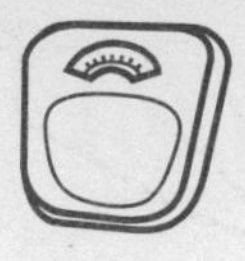

you don't have time to cook, the fresh soups from supermarket chilled cabinets are a good option.

If you live as a family don't say a word about a new regime of eating: just introduce healthier stuff slowly and without comment. If you go in making big statements about eating more healthily they're bound to resist, especially teenagers and men who don't like to be told what to do. Start them off with home-made burgers, thick-cut chips and a really good salad. That'll impress them. Fruit salad for dessert and you're there.

Forget the soft drinks or drastically cut them down. If you have young children don't even let them try it – they're so sweet they'll develop the taste before you know it. The huge calorific intake with each can is thought to be one of the reasons that children are so overweight today.

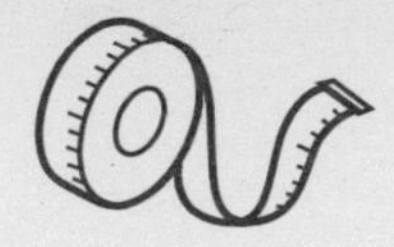

Learn to cook

By learning to cook properly and produce tasty and strong flavours, you can turn even an innocent – and boring-looking – pile of veg into something you really want to eat.

Low-fat chicken curry

If you or your bloke can't go without a curry, which are notoriously high in fat, try this recipe.

4 chicken breasts cut into bite-sized pieces
1 large onion finely chopped
200g veg (could be broccoli, cauliflower, beans, peas)
2 cloves crushed garlic
2 chillies, or more if you like it hot
1–2 tablespoons curry powder
100ml veg stock (from cube is fine)

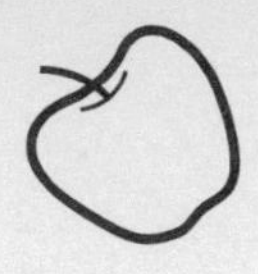

2.5cm piece grated fresh ginger
handful fresh coriander

In a large non stick pan or wok fry the chicken breast until brown (use a little oil if you like). Add onion and veg followed by the garlic, chillies and curry powder. Mix and lower heat, then add stock followed by grated ginger.

Stir well and cover for 15 mins on a low heat. Add more stock if needed. Just before serving throw in the roughly chopped coriander.

If you make it a day or a few hours in advance the flavours will blend and become more intense.

Variation: You can also try this with salmon or cod.

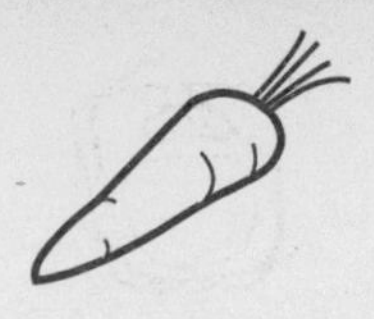

Whenever I go out shopping it is always an absolute killer not to buy chocolate and biscuits ...

You've heard it before, but it really does work: eat before you go out shopping. If you shop on an empty stomach you'll be bound to reach for carbohydrate-loaded grub as it so easily satisfies hunger.

If you don't get a chance to eat before you leave home, grab a fresh smoothie from the cool cabinet, smile at the security man and drink it as you shop.

Take a list with you and stick to it; the only exceptions are fruit and veg, and healthy foods.

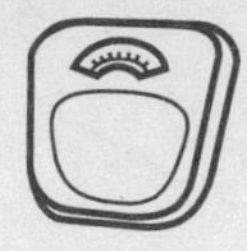

Home-made smoothie

Whiz together a banana, some strawberries or raspberries and a cupful of soya or cow's milk. If you like them a little creamier add a spoonful of yogurt. And if you need some extra fibre you could also add a teaspoon of wheat germ.

I don't feel happy unless I stuff myself at every meal.

Save the stuffing for Christmas Day. The only day in the year when stuffing to bursting point is permitted. In fact it is our duty to eat that way at Christmas.

You've then just got to go for lots of wintry walks to burn off the turkey and pud. How else are you going to fit into those bargains you're going to get in the January sales?

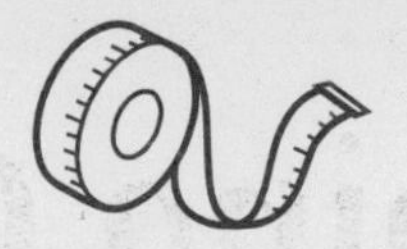

Snacks with drinks! Impossible when I'm trying to watch my weight but my mates need something to nibble on while they're waiting for dinner. What to do ...

Stay away from the peanuts and crisps – every little handful that you throw into your mouth will cost you bigtime at 300 calories a throw.

A handful of peanuts = 300 cals. (Who stops at one? Do the maths: 2 handfuls are 600 cals, almost half a dieting girly's daily intake.)

Instead go for foods that are free, meaning that like a guinea pig eating an entire lettuce you'll probably explode before you'd put on weight from eating them. You can have crudités by the bucketful with a home-made low-fat dip. Pickled onions and baby gherkins are tasty, crunchy and absolutely fine to eat when you really want a snack.

Going Out

Dinner parties

Diplomacy is the keyword. Remember, someone has spent ages cooking for you (unless it's a ready meal, and they're not cheap) so don't blather on about your diet.

If there are things you don't want to eat, have second helpings of the food that won't pile on the weight. Then either leave what you don't want, discreetly, or refuse graciously: 'That looks really fab but I'm completely full up; the ****** was so amazing and I ate so much of it ...' You could offer to collect the plates so that she won't notice that you didn't finish.

Don't let the sight of the choc pud your host has slaved over send you off into a long boring rave about your diet. No one really cares except your host and she'll be offended – or if she's smart realise that there'll be more for the others ...

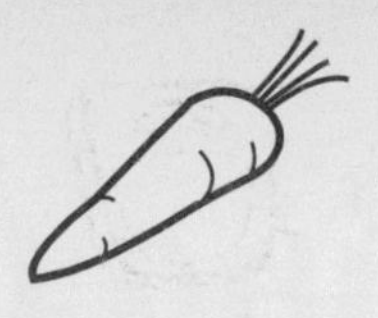

Going to restaurants

Don't get stressed. Enjoy yourself. If you've eaten really well all week, have a day off and indulge yourself.

If you need to stick to your new eating plan, because you've eaten a silly amount, don't make a fuss or draw attention to yourself. Don't bang on about food all evening, making yourself miserable and others bored ... Order something delicious but just not full of butter or cream or loaded with carbs.

To start: Choose the soup – avoiding creamy soups and going for clear vegetable and tomato. Foods with a high water content are filling, so soup before the main meal will lessen your appetite for what follows. (You may even be able to say no to pudding.)

Or choose a fab salad of leaves, tomato and avocado (have the dressing on the side). If you really want the Niçoise ask for it without the deep-fried croutons.

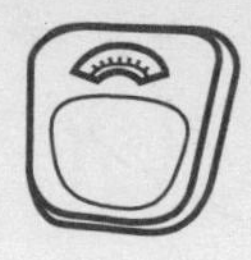

Main course: Choose strong, vibrant-tasting food so that you don't feel deprived: fish, prawns or chicken with chilli, garlic, or herbs like coriander and basil.

Puddings: You can have pudding without blowing it: have the sorbet or fruit.

Got to have the chocolate dessert? If you really must have it, think portion control and ask for a smaller piece. Or share it with someone – equal portions!

- Sauces and dressings – ask for them on the side; eat half only.
- You're in the clear with rice, fish and tomato-based sauces.
- Don't starve yourself before you go out; you'll be more likely to order something sensible if you're not ravenous.
- Keep your hand out of the bread basket – one piece will do.
- Don't talk while you're eating; totally savour every single mouthful.

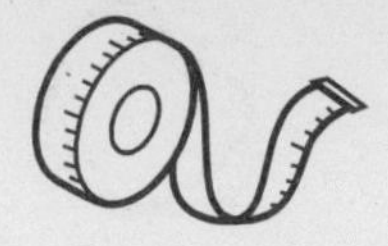

Here's a quick guide to popular restaurant food:

Chinese

- Have the plain, not fried, rice. Crispy duck is delicious but saturated in fat. When you have dim sum choose steamed rather than fried.
- Rice noodles are the best choice with seafood or chicken.
- Forget satay sauce as the peanut base is high in fat.
- Have the steamed spring rolls rather than the fried, they're fresher and tastier too.

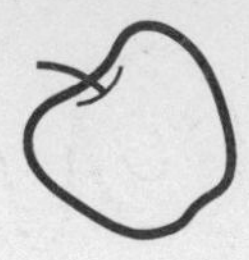

Italian

- Have melon and Parma ham to start, delicious and not too high in fat and cals. There are always loads of meat and fish dishes on the menu and they usually do good salads.
- The best things to choose are the tomato-based dishes: veal or chicken without the breadcrumbs.
- Best to stay away from pasta (vegetarian pastas tend to be the worst choice as they have loads of cheese). You can always have pasta at home, so eat something more exciting.
- Don't have pizza too often – with all that cheese and bread it is quite fattening.

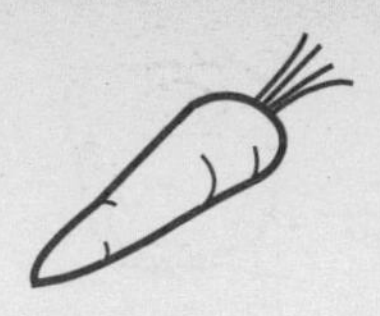

French

- The French are well known for using loads of butter and cream in their cooking.
- Steer clear of confit: confited duck tastes delicious but it is so high in fat and cals.
- You can eat fish, which is often cooked in delicate herbs and white wine. Or bouillabaisse, which is a stunning fish soup.

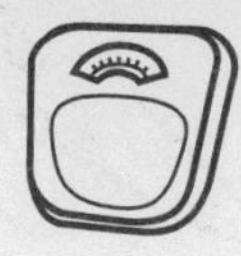

Thai

- Anything fried should be avoided: pad Thai for instance.
- The coconut milk-based dishes are high in fat, as is satay sauce
- The tangy salads, beef for instance, are perfect as are the clear soups like tom yum. Most of the fish dishes should be fine (except the fried ones) and they usually come with a gorgeous sweet chilli sauce for dipping.
- Chicken with basil is also ideal.

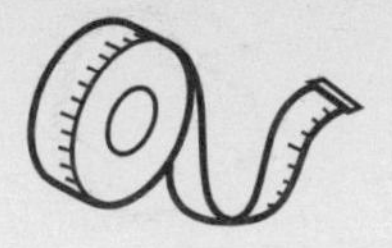

Japanese

- It's pretty easy to eat well, if you avoid the tempura and fried noodles. The sushi, sashimi and clear noodle soups are fab and just what you should be eating.

Spanish

- Tortilla, paella and most tapas are all good – just make sure you don't go for the tapas that are smothered in oil. Olive oil is great stuff but you still have to watch how much you have if you are overweight.

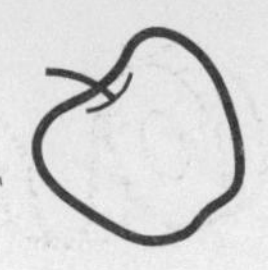

Anti-kebab strategy

Whenever we go out for a drink after work, I'm starving by closing time and always end up wolfing down a greasy kebab ...

Make sure you eat just before you go out for a drink. Pick up something at lunchtime to eat just before you go out, even if it's just a bread roll and cheese, paté, a banana or apple or a ready-made salad from M&S.

A kebab eaten every Friday and Saturday night will result in a substantial weight gain over a year. They're usually disgusting too, and you probably won't even remember having eaten it.

Of course there is the chance you'll contract food poisoning, in which case the pounds will fall away as you lie clutching your stomach in agony.

DON'T TRY THIS AT HOME!

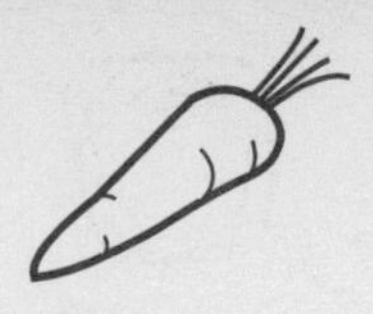

I only ate a sandwich ...

It's up to you to know what you're eating. You may think 'all I ate yesterday was cereal, a salad and a sandwich' – it sounds angelic until you realise what may have been in it.

Sandwich fillings to avoid:

- egg and tuna mayonnaise
- coleslaw

Other pitfalls – Mints, chewing gum, cough lozenges, gravies, ketchup, sauces, dressings, alcohol, thickeners such as flour or cornflour, sugar, salt, oils, butter, margarine, and balsamic vinegar which contains sugar.

You don't need to be obsessive – again the key is always knowing what you're eating so that you are in control. It soon becomes second nature, and then you can relax and forget it.

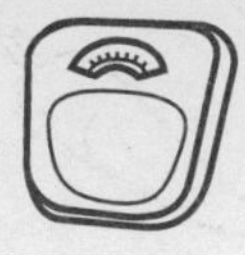

I'll just have a salad ...

Dangers can lurk in your oh-so-innocent-looking salad:

- dressing often contains sugar and salt
- mayonnaise
- croutons – deep fried
- cheese – even shavings of cheese add to the calories
- crispy bacon bits – probably fried, add a lot of cals

Avoid ready-made dressings altogether and make your own simple dressing. If you are eating out, ask for olive oil and vinegar to be brought to the table, so you can put the amount you want on your salad.

Avocado is fine – it is fat, yes, but it is still OK as it's healthy.

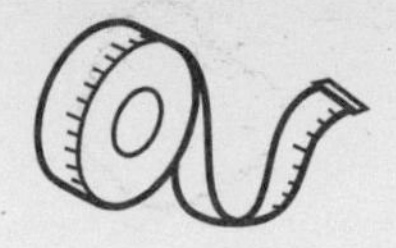

Drinks

A seriously sinister way of piling on the pounds is through your seemingly innocent liquid intake.

The good and the bad news about coffee

The good news: a cup of coffee before exercise will help you to lose weight. Tests on cyclists showed that those who sipped cola or coffee while riding were able to pedal longer and faster than those who drank water. They were able to do 30 per cent more exercise.

The bad news: if you're drinking caffeine (this includes tea and cola) excessively it can affect your blood sugar levels, causing them to drop and making you crave sugar. No more than 2–3 cups a day.

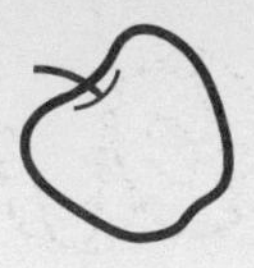

What about my morning cappucino treat?

All of the 'American-style coffee chains' have introduced enormously decadent coffee treats including mochas and hot chocolate. Piled with cream and topped with chocolate they can 'sneak' up to 300+ calories into your system when you think the worst you're doing is having a caffeine fix to get you going.

You can't even escape in the summer as they now serve chilled, iced-coffee combos to tempt you.

To make things worse, if you just happen to grab one of the little chocolate treats, or cookies enticingly displayed on the counter, you'll really pile on the weight while kidding yourself you're just having morning coffee.

The fact that you're not properly awake yet is no excuse!

A plain white coffee is the lowest in calories followed by cappuccino, latte and, worst of all, hot chocolate. If you ask for the low-fat milk option the cals will be lower.

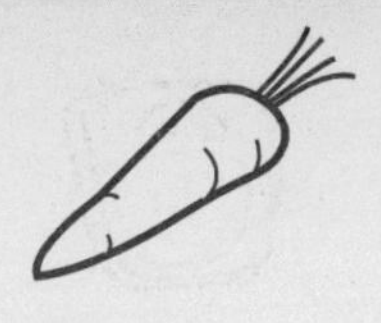

Booze and your body

I know it's fun and a big part of your social life but you might need to look at what you drink and how much you drink. The truth is that booze bloats you and the calories it contains are 'empty', that is it has no nutritional value.

An American study has shown that drinking less than 3 units per day did not lead to weight gain; more than this and weight shot up.

You probably don't want to give it up but it's worth knowing which type of bevvies are lower in calories and which ones you should stay away from.

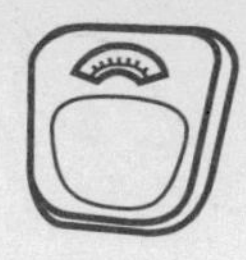

What should I drink when I'm out?

This list will help you decide

Lowest to highest in calorie content:

Baileys 25ml 80 cals
vodka 25ml 50 cals
gin & tonic 25ml 55 cals
champagne 125ml 95 cals
small glass of wine, 115ml: red 70 cals, white 65 cals
1/2 of most lagers, 120 cals
bottle of Diamond White 145 cals
Bacardi Breezer 180 cals

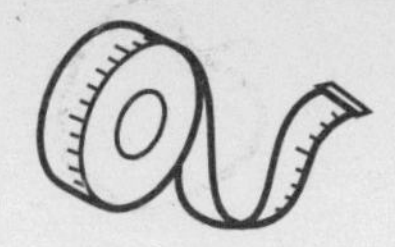

Calorie-saving tip:

Halve your wine calories by drinking spritzers instead of all wine. If you have 50% wine and 50% soda you'll save calories for something else. Soda has no calories so you're talking 35 cals for a spritzer (60ml wine) instead of 70 cals for a glass of wine (120ml)

This works for red wine, as well as white, and is really refreshing in the summer as it chills the wine a little.

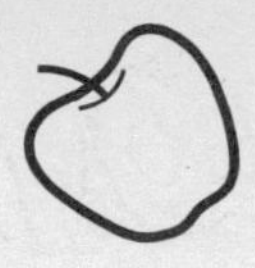

Are Alcopops okay?

Sugar, sugar, sugar. You can tell just by how sticky the bottle gets when you're holding it that these drinks are seriously high in sugar. They scream calories!

They go straight to your head and your waist simultaneously. 180 cals per drink as opposed to a bottle of cider which is 145 and a vodka tonic which is 50 cals.

Your best bet is a single shot of spirit like gin or vodka with a tonic or cranberry mixer – definitely not cola or lemonade.

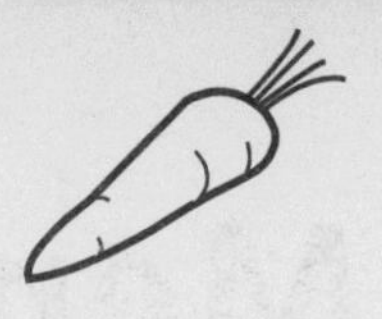

Girls' night out

Lager … Lager … LARGER!

Find a lower-fat tipple than lager – always go for wine rather than beer. Apart from the calories, beer is loaded with carbs.

Dancing it off:

A sobering thought: the more wine you drink, the longer you will have to keep dancing to burn off those calories …

Men

Relationships are a mixed blessing when it comes to weight. Getting dumped is likely to set you off on a binge, whether its a whole packet of biscuits or booze. BUT domestic bliss can also make you pile on the pounds, nights spent in front of the TV eating popcorn instead of being out clubbing. Your only hope is to make some effort on the sex front to get in some exercise.

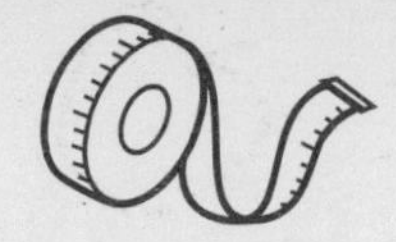

My boyfriend is so mean about my weight

Don't accept constant criticisms. You'll know if you want to lose weight – it's for you to do and for you to decide. The only time blokes are allowed to nag is if you're so overweight that your health is at risk. Then it's not nagging, it's love in action.

Oh my God moments

A passion killer all right: having sex, legs in the air, you suddenly notice your saddlebags – well, roll girl, roll and get on top, things look better from there.

Focus on his fat to make you feel you're not alone.

He's got a six pack? Get yourself a corset with the excuse that it looks super sexy.

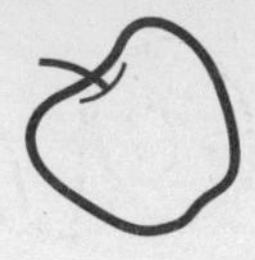

Sexy foods that aren't fattening

- champagne (this may be a lie but it makes sense to believe it)
- yoghurt poured onto you for your lover to lick off – actually, seeing as he's the one doing the licking and consuming the calories why not make it chocolate?
- oysters
- a ripe, juicy mango – eaten with someone equally luscious in bed
- strawberries

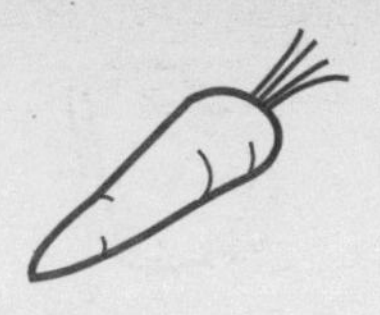

My boyfriend teases me a lot about my weight and makes 'fat' jokes, it really winds me up ...

Don't let him get away with it. Ask him why he does it. If he's typical of a lot of blokes he'll say 'it's just a joke', but he may realise that it really upsets you and stop.

A good technique is not to react or even sulk, just leave the room whenever he does it as if you're going to get something. Consciously or subconsciously he'll get the message.

Never, ever tell fat jokes at your own expense ... Don't let people have you pinned down as the fat lady.

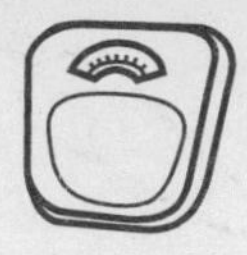

Reasons not to overeat:
A large meal before sex will make you feel tired and bloated. Keep it light and stay sexy.

My man also needs to lose weight but he just won't listen ...

Appeal to the macho man in him. Get your bloke to show you his football or rugby-training warm-ups. They're good fun and probably a lot different from anything you've ever done before. If he's a tennis or golf freak then ask him for some coaching. Most men love to tell someone how to do things so here's his big chance. Get yourself a really funky tracksuit that you look fab in and enjoy it. It's a really fun and sneaky way of enticing him to get fit without him knowing it.

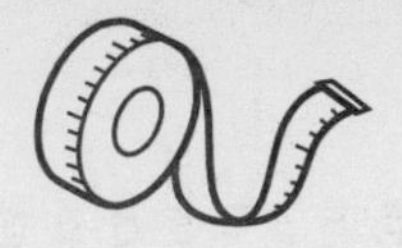

My man has to have his pasta with his meal every night …

- If he's not part of the solution, he's part of the problem. If he insists on eating crap food, don't go down with him, or rather, up in size.
- If he cooks just leave the pasta and don't eat it, not more than once a week anyway. If you cook, find some seriously tasting but calorie-conscious recipes so that he won't notice the difference. If he complains you will just have to put your foot down, when *you* cook, you cook what you want to cook.

Glam incentive

If he's keen for you to lose weight then get him to help (and put his money where his mouth is) by promising you a glam designer outfit when you reach the size you want to be.

Conclusion

Making changes in your life won't always be easy, so be prepared for bad days and always have a recovery plan for the day after. If you eat that cake and fall off your new way of eating just treat it as a temporary glitch and get back on track as soon as you can. Phone a friend, get some encouragement to keep on eating the right way to lose weight.

Always eat on time: eat before you get really hungry as that is when you'll be in danger of eating the wrong thing or gobbling up a whole packet of biscuits. Always have loads of the right things in your cupboards and freezer and get rid of all the rubbishy stuff.

Stop eating before you feel full and stuffed – the only excuse for this is Christmas, though all it does is to make you feel fit for nothing but the rest of the afternoon in front of the box.

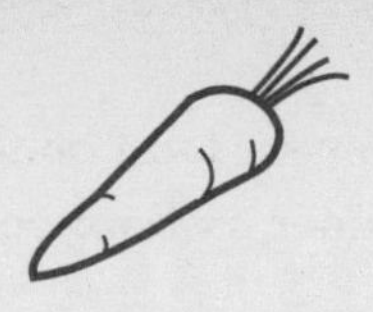

Focus on attacking your weaknesses to stop them undermining your weight loss. Do cut out the bad carbs, cakes and biscuits, croissants and too much pasta. And steer clear of processed, frozen and ready-made foods. Watch that you're not living on fatty foods – remember to have the good fats but avoid chips and pizza or any other fast food.

Find the exercise that is right for you whether it's aerobics, sex or clubbing. Don't force yourself into doing something you hate. If all else fails go for regular brisk walks, go with a friend and make them a social occasion.

Make all of this a habit, a permanent lifestyle change, and you'll soon be looking in the mirror at a glam new you.

Happy eating!

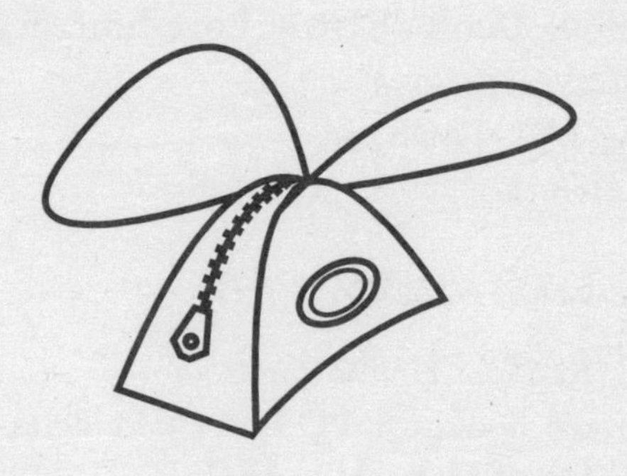